QUALITATIVE RESEARCH METHODS IN SPORT, EXERCISE AND HEALTH

The qualitative method is perhaps the most dynamic and exciting area of contemporary research in sport, exercise and health. Students and researchers at all levels are now expected to understand qualitative approaches and to employ these in their work. In this comprehensive introductory text, Andrew C. Sparkes and Brett Smith take the reader on a journey through the research process, offering a guide to the fundamentals of qualitative research.

Each chapter contains comprehensive knowledge to enable new researchers to engage with and experience core methods and procedures, from semi-structured interviews to content analysis. The book also explores the 'what', 'when' and 'how' questions within all of the central traditions within qualitative research. For example, what is ethnography? When might it be appropriate to use an ethnographic approach, and how does one conduct an ethnographic study? Each chapter is also vividly illustrated with cases and examples from real research in sport, exercise and health. The book also goes further than any other textbook in exploring innovative contemporary methods, such as visual and sensual ethnography.

Qualitative Research Methods in Sport, Exercise and Health is essential reading for any student, researcher or professional working on a research project in a sport, exercise or health context.

Andrew C. Sparkes is Professor of Sport, Physical Activity and Leisure at Leeds Metropolitan University, UK.

Brett Smith is Reader in Qualitative Health Research in the Peter Harrison Centre for Disability Sport at Loughborough University, UK. He is Editor-in-Chief of the journal *Qualitative Research in Sport, Exercise and Health*.

From Andrew: To my Mum, Dad, Kitty, Jessica and Alexander – for everything and forever.

From Brett: To Cassie with love, admiration and excitement about adventures that lie ahead.

QUALITATIVE RESEARCH METHODS IN SPORT, EXERCISE AND HEALTH

FROM PROCESS TO PRODUCT

ANDREW C. SPARKES AND
BRETT SMITH

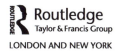

LONDON AND NEW YORK

First published 2014
by Routledge
2 Park Square, Milton Park, Abingdon, Oxon OX14 4RN

Simultaneously published in the USA and Canada
by Routledge
711 Third Avenue, New York, NY 10017

Routledge is an imprint of the Taylor & Francis Group, an informa business

British Library Cataloguing in Publication Data
A catalogue record for this book is available from the British Library

Library of Congress Cataloging in Publication Data
Qualitative research methods in sport, exercise and health :
from product / edited by Andrew C. Sparkes and Brett Smith.
pages cm
1. Sports sciences—Research—Methodology.
2. Exercise—Research—Methodolgy.
Qualitative research—Methodology. I. Sparkes, Andrew C.
GV558.Q35 2014
613.71—dc23
2013012001

ISBN: 978–0–415–57834–9 (hbk)
ISBN: 978–0–415–57835–6 (pbk)
ISBN: 978–0–203–85218–7 (ebk)

Typeset in Melior and Univers
by Swales & Willis Ltd, Exeter, Devon

CONTENTS

INTRODUCTION

In the preface to the third edition of the *Handbook of Qualitative Research*, the editors, Denzin and Lincoln (2005), note that, over the past quarter century, a quiet methodological revolution has been occurring in the social sciences that has led to a growth in qualitative forms of research that 'is nothing short of amazing' (p. ix). Likewise, describing the growth in qualitative research within psychology and across the social and health sciences, Madill and Gough (2009) use the term *phenomenal*. They note that qualitative articles are being published increasingly in mainstream psychology journals, as well as there being an explosion of dedicated textbooks, journals, conferences and workshops attempting to address the demand for qualitative research from students, researchers, practitioners and policy makers.

More recently, in their review of qualitative research published in three leading sports psychology journals during 2000–2009, Culver, Gilbert and Sparkes (2012) point to a 68 percent increase in qualitative studies published since the period 1990–1999 (from 17.3 percent to 29 percent). When examining individual journals, the *Journal of Applied Sport Psychology* more than doubled the percentage of qualitative articles published (16.7–35 percent), *The Sport Psychologist* increased 68 percent (30.3–50.9 percent), and the *Journal of Sport & Exercise Psychology* increased 37 percent (7.5–10.3 percent). Overall there was an increase in the number of qualitative articles published in the three journals by 31.7 percent. Finally, compared with the previous decade, Culver *et al.* note that there is much greater variety in the authors who are publishing qualitative research in these journals. Whereas in the original review 3 researchers were named as authors in 31 of the 84 articles, there was no such dominance in the years 2000–2009. Indeed, in *The Sport Psychologist* where the most qualitative articles were published, only 9 researchers published more than one article as the first author, and 75 different researchers published more than one article not as the first author, and 75 different researchers are first authors of the 85 qualitative articles published (Culver *et al.* 2012).

Apparently then, not only is more qualitative research getting published in these journals but also, very importantly, more scholars are engaging with and producing qualitative work.

Dart (2012) sought to conduct a similar comparison of methodologies used in the *International Review for the Sociology of Sport*, the *Journal of Sport and Social Issues* and the *Sociology of Sport Journal*. He was not, however, able to accomplish this task as the title, abstract and key words for many of the papers in these journals were not clear as to what method(s) had been employed. This said, these journals do support qualitative research as evidenced in their publication record. The same can be said for journals that are multidisciplinary in nature, such as, *Sport, Education and Society*. Against this backdrop, the maturity, scope and challenges associated with qualitative research in recent years acted to support the formulation of a new journal launched in 2009 entitled *Qualitative Research in Sport, Exercise and Health* (Routledge, Taylor and Francis Group) that since its inception has been dedicated to supporting innovative methodologies within a multi-disciplinary framework.

Given this wealth of resources it might appear a good time to be a qualitative researcher. Well, it is and it isn't. While these resources are to be welcomed as a means of providing a secure foundation to build on by those wishing to enter the domain of qualitative inquiry in sport, exercise and health (SEH), the same set of resources can also be bewildering and confusing. This is because, despite its apparent similarities, qualitative research is not just one thing. Rather, qualitative research is many things to different people. Just what qualitative research is, what its purposes are, and how it might be conducted and represented are evolving phenomena. As Walsh and Koelsch (2012) comment:

> If the field of qualitative research is at all a camp, it is a camp compromised of many small communities with distinct languages and traditions. Nevertheless, most of us who inhabit this camp prefer to affirm our common bonds. Yet, underlying these bonds are important distinctions that shape how we think – about research, about knowledge, and about human nature . . . Within traditions, what were once deemed canonical texts and practices are undergoing change, shaped by evolving thought both within and outside of those approaches.
>
> (Walsh & Koelsch, 2012: 380)

2

Our task in this book, therefore, is to introduce some of the communities or traditions that make up the qualitative camp and what holds it together. We also examine some of the differences within and between traditions, which generate creative tensions which in turn stimulate dialogue and lead to change over time. These similarities and differences are deeply connected to issues revolving around the processes involved in the doing of qualitative research and the kinds of products that are generated for public consumption. These processes are closely interwoven and should not be viewed as detached and independent entities in and of themselves. This interweaving informs and shapes what qualitative researchers think, feel and do throughout their study from start to finish.

The similarities that hold the qualitative camp together in terms of its core assumptions and practices, and which make it different from quantitative research, are the focus of Chapter 1. Our task in Chapter 2 is to introduce a selection of the key communities or traditions that are members of the qualitative research camp and to give a flavour of each by discussing their central features whilst also recognising their subtle differences. In Chapter 3 we focus on a number of important pre-study tasks that should be done before data collection and analysis begin in earnest. Accordingly, in Chapter 4 we give an overview of the various methods or techniques that qualitative researchers can use to collect data. These range from the traditional (for example, interviewing) to more novel or emerging methods of data collection (for example, the visual and the Internet). Just as there are a range of data collection techniques for qualitative researchers as *bricoleurs* to draw upon, so it is with the forms of analysis available to them. Chapter 5, therefore, focuses on the main forms of analysis used by researchers in SEH and also considers some emerging forms that are beginning to have an impact.

Having collected the data and analysed it, the findings of a study have to be communicated to others. This is no easy task and poor or inappropriate forms of communication can undermine the efforts of researchers regardless of their good intentions and the importance of the results. In Chapter 6, therefore, we consider a variety of representational forms, ranging from the traditional realist tale to communicating qualitative findings via musical performances. Given that there are multiple ways for qualitative researchers to conceptualise their studies, conduct these, collect data, analyse the data, and then report their findings, questions are raised about how such work, in its various forms and traditions, might be judged. Chapter 7 addresses this question by examining what terms like objectivity, reliability, generalisability and validity might mean in qualitative research, if they mean anything at all. Alternative criteria for passing appropriate judgments on qualitative work in the form of flexible lists are proposed and illustrated in action. It is recommended that in order to make fair and ethical judgements about the work of different research traditions, scholars need to develop the skills and characteristics of the connoisseur.

Part of this connoisseurship involves an appreciation of the ethical dilemmas that qualitative researchers encounter throughout their studies. In Chapter 8, therefore, traditional approaches to ethics are explored and their limitations highlighted prior to considering a range of alternative positions framed by what might be described as an aspirational ethics. The complexities of such ethics in the field as an unfolding process over time are illuminated, and the practical implications of this for qualitative researchers in relation to core issues are discussed in detail. Finally, in Chapter 9 we offer some brief reflections on the necessary art of conceptual self-defence for qualitative researchers along with the requirement for them to become better at educating colleagues, policymakers and other audiences about the benefits their work has in a variety of contexts that range from the local to the international. We suggest there is a need to find new strategic and tactical ways to work with one another in the new paradigm dialogue and consider the potential of transdisciplinary research as one part in this process. We conclude that those who practice qualitative research should take pride in the different kinds of knowledge, understanding and awareness they contribute to SEH and look forward to the dynamic and innovative offerings they will make in the future.

In closing this introduction, we hope that the content, form and sentiments expressed by us in the chapters that follow will be of some interest to readers, even though they might not agree with our stance on key issues and our views on both the processes involved and the products of qualitative research in SEH. We are certainly not saying there is only one way to do qualitative research, or that our way is best, or that other approaches both old and new are 'bad'. Rather, we have put forward our ideas in this book as *one* way to conceptualise the field of qualitative research and go about practicing this form of inquiry. It is simply an approach we have found useful in our own work, as have our undergraduate and postgraduate students on the courses we teach, and who are our harshest critics and ask the toughest questions. We are forever in their debt.

4

As with any volume of this kind, we have had to be selective about what issues to include and whose work to cite as exemplars. We are, therefore, necessarily guilty of the charges of exclusion and omission and we have felt the weight of these charges in putting the book together. For those, whose excellent work has not been included, we apologise. Importantly, for those whose work we have included we hope we have done justice to their scholarship. The ever-present failures in the text are entirely ours.

CHAPTER 1

WHAT IS QUALITATIVE RESEARCH?

Just as there is no clear-cut and unanimously agreed definition of *quantitative* research so it is with *qualitative* research. For Avis (2005), 'almost every aspect of qualitative research, what it is, what it is for, how it is done, and how it is to be judged, is the subject of controversy' (p. 3). At best, the label 'qualitative research' is an umbrella term to describe a camp compromised of many small communities with distinct languages and traditions (Walsh & Koelsch, 2012). Having reviewed developments in qualitative research over the last twenty five years, Lincoln (2010) describes the current position as follows:

> We are interpretivists, postmodernists, poststructuralists; we are phenomenological, feminist, critical. We choose lenses that are border, racial, ethnic, hybrid, queer, differently abled, indigenous, margin, center, Other. Fortunately, qualitative research – with or without the signifiers – has been porous, permeable, and highly assimilative. Its practitioners, adherents, and theorists have come from multiple disciplines and have brought to the project of qualitative invention the literatures, philosophies, disciplinary stances, and professional commitments of the social sciences, medicine, nursing, communication studies, social welfare, fisheries, wildlife, tourism, and a dozen other academic specialities. Consequently, we have acquired richness and elaboration that has both added to our confusion and at the same time, been broad and pliant enough to encompass a variety of claimants.
>
> (p. 8)

Not surprisingly, Denzin and Lincoln (2005) emphasise that there is no *one* way to do qualitative inquiry and speak of multiple interpretive projects. Likewise, Madill and Gough (2009) argue that the situation in the early twenty-first century is one of heterogeneity, with qualitative research best conceptualised as a fuzzy set. For them,

6

the field consists of clusters of methods with features in common that overlap, in some respect with other clusters, while at the same time, some methods have no obvious features in common with other methods. To complicate matters further, because qualitative methods can be clustered in different ways, no typology is definitive.

(p. 255)

Given these problems of definition, it is interesting to note how both quantitative and qualitative research are often defined by virtue of what these are *not* and placed in opposition to the 'other' via the use of socially constructed dichotomies (that is, mutually exclusive, paired opposites) such as art/science, hard/soft and numbers/words. For Martin (2011), articles examining quantitative and qualitative research frequently highlight and over-emphasise the difference between these two approaches. He suggests, 'differences are typically portrayed as dichotomous vs. differences in emphasis or degree. Additionally, similarities and shared middle ground are often ignored' (p. 335). This can lead to incomplete, inaccurate and misleading reviews on both types of research that does not do justice to the contributions each makes to our understanding of the world around us. That said, Martin acknowledges that there *are* areas of legitimate and substantial *difference* between quantitative and qualitative research that need to be considered.

Outlining legitimate and substantial differences between quantitative and qualitative is part of our task in this chapter. In so doing, we by necessity identify some of the commonalities and basic methodological premises that hold the qualitative camp together (see Chapter 2). Such commonalities (even though they might be contested) provide a starting point for discussions about the nature of qualitative research in general and what craft and way of being can offer those interested in better understanding the domains of sport, exercise and health (SEH). Likewise, recognising common differences between qualitative and quantitative research provides a starting point for conversations about what each approach has to offer each other and the field of SEH in terms of the different forms of knowing about phenomena these provide.

In what follows, therefore, we draw upon *ideal types* of qualitative and quantitative research. An ideal type is a *construct* that is a description of a phenomenon in its abstract form. These do not exist in pure form. However, ideal types are useful in assisting researchers to compare and classify phenomenon. For example, consider how Gubrium and Holstein (1997) use this strategy in comparing the 'methods talk' of two different kinds of sociologists working in the same faculty. One group are quantitative researchers, who treat social facts as things, and then attempt to measure these with the aim of describing and explaining their relationships via a highly technical language. There is talk of structural variables and causal models, units of analysis and sampling frames, operationalisation and measurement, cluster analysis and multidimensional scaling, stochastic processes, multicolinearity, and autocorrelation. In contrast, at the other end of the corridor are a smaller group of qualitative researchers who are easily identified by talk that seems more *experientially* poignant.

> There's lots of talk about *meaning*, especially about what things mean to the people being studied. This is decidedly not talk about predictive models. *Lived* experience is on stage here. Rich description is the name of the game. There's little mention of standardised measurement. Instead we hear the trials and tribulations of 'entre and engagement,' 'access and rapport.' In contrast to descriptions of social facts and variable relations from an 'objective' distance – held at arm's length so to speak – we hear the admonition to get close to people, be involved. 'You've got to get out there, into the nitty-gritty, real world. Get your hands dirty. See it up close, for yourself.'
>
> (Gubrium & Holstein, 1997: 4)

Many will recognise these ideal types in action. Indeed, in a special edition of *Qualitative Research in Sport, Exercise and Health* (2011, Volume 3, No. 2) that was devoted to quantitative researchers' views of qualitative research (see for example Hagger & Chatzisarantis, 2011; Latimer, Martin-Ginis & Perrier, 2011; Eklund, Jeffery, Dobersek & Cho, 2011; Horn, 2011; Gill, 2011; Scanlan, 2011; Berry, 2011; Brewer, Vose, Van Raalte & Pepetitpas, 2011; Martin, 2011), a number of contributions reflect these different worlds of meaning making in action as they explore the possibilities of dialogue between the two. We can, therefore, draw on ideal types as a heuristic device to consider some of the general *characteristics* of qualitative and quantitative research. The next section examines the philosophical assumptions and methodological commitments that inform, but do not determine, how qualitative and quantitative researchers go about their work. This is called the *paradigms* approach. Following this, we consider the key characteristics of qualitative researcher in terms of what its practitioners actually *do* when they conduct their studies. This is called the *practical* approach.

THE PARADIGMS APPROACH

> Paradigms and metaphysics *do* matter. They matter because they tell us something important about *researcher standpoint.* They tell us something about the researcher's proposed *relationship to the Other(s).* They tell us something about what the researcher thinks *counts as knowledge*, and *who can deliver the most valuable slice of this knowledge.* They tell us how the researcher intends to *take account of multiple and contradictory values* she will encounter.
>
> (Lincoln, 2010: 7, emphasis in original)

A paradigm, according to Guba and Lincoln (1994: 107), is a 'set of *basic beliefs* (or metaphysics) . . . and a *worldview* that defines, for its holder, the nature of the "world", the individual's place in it, and the range of possible relationships to that world and its parts'. The basic beliefs, assumptions and postulates of a paradigm are learned via the processes of socialisation, telling researchers what is important, legitimate and reasonable to study. Paradigms are also normative, in that paradigms tell researchers what and how to do things with little need for reflection on questions such as: Why are things done this way? This is both the strength and the weakness of paradigms. They make action possible but the very reasons for the action are hidden in the unquestioned assumptions of the paradigm. This forms a mutually self-reinforcing process. That is, we conduct inquiry via a particular paradigm because it embodies assumptions about the world that we believe in and supports values that we hold dear. And, because we hold those assumptions and values we conduct inquiry according to the precepts of that paradigm.

This comment would seem to challenge the view that the research 'problem' or question constitutes the first step in any study and thereafter drives it. Here, the 'problem' or research question should define the approach and methods used. It could, however, be argued that people are attracted to and shape research 'problems' that match their personal way of seeing and understanding the world. That is, it is not the research 'problem' or question that drives a study, but, either implicitly or explicitly, our assumptions and theoretical orientations. Gill (2011), speaking as a self-defined 'non-qualitative' researcher, notes that the question–method relationship is more complicated than simply stating that the question should drive the method.

> Questions set our destination, but they often also set the direction or path. Questions do not arise out of thin air. Rather our questions come from us (the researchers) and are influenced by a host of factors including our training, experiences, and immediate surroundings. Many of us are already well down the path of quantitative research (even in graduate school); we know the landmarks, pitfalls, shortcuts, and we have made good progress – we cannot just turn around and wander off into the woods.
>
> (Gill, 2011: 309)

The issues raised by Gill (2011) relate to how researchers respond to the questions posed by the basic beliefs of a paradigm. For Denzin and Lincoln (2005: 22) these include the following; 'beliefs about ontology (What kind of being is the human being? What is the nature of reality?), epistemology (What is the relationship between the inquirer and the known?), and methodology (How do we know the world or gain knowledge of it?)'.

At a fundamental level, researchers of different paradigmatic persuasions respond to these questions in different ways. Krane and Baird (2005) provide a review of the foundational positions and assumptions of what they see as the major contemporary research paradigms. They then compare each paradigm in terms of its position with regard to the nature of knowledge, the goal of inquiry, the role of values, the role of theory, the way in which voice is represented, the researcher role, and the criteria used to judge the legitimacy of the research. Their comparisons illustrate how key *differences* operate between researchers and their named paradigms.

For example, the researcher's role within quantitative research is that of 'disinterested scientist'. In contrast, for the constructivist (that is, qualitative researcher) the same role becomes that of 'passionate participant'. With regard to the nature of knowledge, both social constructionists and critical theorists agree that there are multiple realities in operation but disagree about the goals of inquiry and the researcher role. The goal of inquiry for the social constructionist is 'understanding the natural setting' whereas for the critical theorist it's about 'empowerment and emancipation' and the researcher's role is that of a 'transformative intellectual' who operates as an advocate and an activist (also see Guba & Lincoln, 2005; Martin, 2011; Chapter 2 this volume). Such comparisons confirm, there *are* differences that *do* make a difference when it comes to paradigmatic thinking both within and between paradigms. It would be foolish to ignore them. For our purposes, and at the risk of gross simplification, we will now compare some of the key paradigmatic differences between quantitative and qualitative researchers as ideal types.

Regarding the ontological question, quantitative researchers adhere to a *realist* or *external* view of reality. This assumes that a single, uniform and objective reality exists externally 'out there' and independent from the person. This reality imposes itself on individual consciousness from without and is driven by immutable natural laws and mechanisms that are apprehendable. The aim of research, therefore, is to formulate rules beyond time and space in order to control and predict. As Guba and Lincoln (1994: 109) state: 'Knowledge of the "way things are" is conventionally summarised in the form of time- and context-free generalisations, some of which take the form of cause–effect laws. Research can, in principle, converge on the true state of affairs.'

Addressing the ontological question, qualitative researchers adopt a *relativist or internal* ontology. This conceives of social reality as humanly constructed and shaped in ways that make it fluid and multifaceted. Multiple, subjective realities exist in the form of mental constructions. In this perspective it *is* accepted that physical things exist out there independent of ourselves. However, as Smith (1989) notes, the mind plays a foundational role in the shaping or constructing of social reality, and therefore what exists 'is not independent of, but in a very significant sense is dependent on our minds' (p. 74). This does not mean that the mind 'creates' the world of objects or what people say or do. Rather, it means that how we give meaning to objects and how we interpret the movements and utterances of other people, in terms of the motivations and meanings we assign to them, are shaped by the determining categories of the mind via, for example, language and cultural symbolism.

Guba and Lincoln (1994) argue that realities are apprehended in the form of intangible mental constructions, 'socially and experientially based, local and specific in nature (although elements are often shared among many individuals and even across cultures), and dependent for their form and content on the individual persons or group holding the constructions' (p. 111). The constructions that people hold, therefore, are alterable, as are their associated 'realities'. More recently, these points are echoed in Gubrium and Holstein's (2008) description of *constructionism* in which 'the leading idea always has been that the world we live in and our place in it are not simply and evidently "there" for participants. Rather, participants actively construct the world of everyday life and its constituent elements' (p. 3). This point is well illustrated by Dingwell (1992) in his reflections on the notion of disease.

> This point is important in understanding the boundaries between social and natural scientific studies in medicine. There are no diseases in nature, merely relationships between organisms . . . Diseases are produced by the conceptual schemes imposed on the natural world by human beings, which value some states of the body and disvalue others. This is not to say that biological changes may not impose themselves on us, but rather that the significance of those changes depends upon their location in human society. The normal physiology of ageing is relevant in very different ways to an East African herdsman who sees it as a mark of advancing status, power and sexual attractiveness and to a Californian actress who sees it as the beginning of her decline as a social being.
>
> (p. 165)

For the qualitative researcher, multifaceted, constructed realities exist and the process of inquiry is a matter of interpreting the interpretations of others. The aim of research is to focus on the particular ways in which people construct their meanings of a given phenomenon, seeking to expand the understanding of the phenomenon through the individual case. The job of qualitative researchers, therefore, is to acknowledge and report these different realities by relying on the voices and interpretations of the participants through extensive quotes, presenting themes that reflect the words and actions of participants, and advancing evidence of different perspectives on each theme (Creswell, 2007).

Regarding *epistemological* issues and questions concerning the nature of the relationship between the knower or would-be knower and those involved in the study, quantitative researchers adopt a *dualist* and *objectivist* position. This assumes that the researcher and the researched 'object' are independent entities, and the researcher is capable of studying the object without influencing it or being influenced by it. That is, the knower can stand outside of what is to be known, values can be sus-

12

pended in order to understand, and 'true objectivity' (or something very close to it) is possible as long as the researcher adopts a distant, detached, non-interactive posture (as if looking at the world through a one-way mirror). It is assumed that theory-free knowledge and observation can be achieved. To avoid the potential dangers of values introducing 'bias' to the proceedings, quantitative researchers advocate the use of prescribed technical procedures to reduce or eliminate such influence.

In contrast, qualitative researchers propose a *subjectivist, transactional and constructionist* epistemology. What is studied is not 'out there' independent of inquirers. On the contrary, inquirers, Smith (1989) points out, both in their day-to-day lives and as professionals, are thoroughly and inseparably a part of what is studied. This is often described as a subject–subject relationship as opposed to a subject–object dualism. From this epistemological position, there can be no separation of the researcher and the researched, and values *always* mediate and shape what is understood. The knower and the known are inter-dependent and fused together in such a way that the 'findings' are the creation of a process of interaction between the two. As such, there can be no theory-free knowledge.

The difference between qualitative and quantitative researchers in how they answer the questions about ontology and epistemology actively influence how they develop their *methodologies*. Quantitative researchers who adhere to a realist ontology and a dualist or objectivist epistemology, and whose purpose is to explain, predict and control phenomena, tend to favour an *experimental* and *manipulative* approach. Here, questions and/or hypotheses are stated in propositional form and subjected to empirical testing to verify or falsify these under carefully controlled and manipulated conditions. There is a heavy reliance on increasingly sophisticated forms of statistical analysis to interpret the data generated which is normally numerical in nature.

In contrast, qualitative researchers who hold a relativist ontology, a subjectivist, transactional and constructionist epistemology, and whose purpose is to understand and interpret the world from the participants' point of view, favour a *hermeneutical* and *dialectical* approach. This is described by Guba and Lincoln (1994) as follows.

> The variable and personal (intramental) nature of social constructions suggest that individual constructions can be elicited and refined only through interactions *between* and *among*

investigator and respondents. These varying constructions are interpreted using conventional hermeneutical techniques and are compared and contrasted through dialectical interchange.

(p. 111)

The basic philosophical differences as we have described them, lead to quantitative and qualitative researchers developing different research designs, using different techniques to collect different kinds of data, performing different types of analyses, representing their findings in different ways, and judging the 'quality' of their studies using different criteria. These differences are important to recognise and acknowledge. For some, these differences are problematic. For us, however, such differences are to be celebrated and valued because they allow us to know and understand the world of SEH in diverse and enriched ways.

THE PRACTICAL APPROACH

Looking at the philosophical assumptions that inform and guide qualitative research is a very useful way of getting a sense of what holds this camp together. Another way is to examine what qualitative researchers from various traditions actually *do*, or say they do, in action so as to reveal the common characteristics or threads that bind them together. The following are a few that we have identified in the literature.

Focus on meanings, subjectivity, context and process

Qualitative research is a form of social inquiry that focuses on the way people interpret and make sense of their experiences and the world in which they live. Most of the traditions within it have the same aim, which is, to understand the social reality of individuals, groups and cultures, and explore the behaviours, perspectives and experiences of people in their daily lives. Charmaz (2004) points out that we *enter* the phenomenon to discover what is significant from the viewpoints and actions of people who experience it in relation to time, place, context and situation – and people. For her, the task is to learn the logic of the experiences we study and not simply to impose our logic on it. It is through the process of learning this logic that the meanings and actions of the participants become clearer to us.

14

Besides gathering the overt meanings that people express, Charmaz (2004) notes how qualitative research celebrates discovering the take-for-granted meanings that inform their actions which, for the most part, are tacit, liminal and implicit.

> To appreciate what is happening in a setting, we need to know what it means to participants. Meanings render action and intention comprehensible. Actions can make implicit meanings visible. We observe our research participants grappling with making sense of their lives, and then we grapple with them trying to do so.
>
> (Charmaz, 2004: 981)

For Gubrium and Holstein (1997), 'a world comprised of meanings, interpretations, feelings, talk, and interaction must be scrutinised on its own terms' (p. 13). Therefore, the topic of *subjectivity* is paramount for qualitative researchers who seek to explore the multiple meanings that people attach to their experiences, and who then identify and describe the social structures and processes that shape these meanings. They try to capture social events from the perspective of those involved in them, to provide an insider's view of social life, by 'walking in their shoes' to better understand what and how they feel in making sense of the world around them.

> Entering the phenomenon means being fully present during the interview and deep inside the content afterward. Not only does this focused attention validate your participant's humanity, it also helps you to take a close look at what you are gaining. Entering the phenomenon means that you come to sense, feel, and fathom what having this experience is like, although you enter your participants' lives much less than an ethnographer. Entering the phenomenon also means that your active involvement with data shapes the analysis. A few descriptive codes and a powerful computer program do not suffice.
>
> (Charmaz, 2004: 981)

This 'entering into' is often described as an *emic* perspective. This is concerned with the quality and texture of experience, along with its dynamics and development as a process over time, rather than with the identification of cause–effect relationships. Qualitative researchers, therefore, tend not to work with 'variables' that are defined by the researcher before the research process begins. This is because they are interested in the meaning attributed to events by the participants themselves. Using preconceived 'variables' would lead to the imposition of the researcher's meanings and it would preclude the identification of respondents' own ways of making sense of the phenomenon under investigation.

Regarding the emic perspective, in his study of bodybuilding, drugs and risk, Monaghan (2001) states that 'as a qualitative study, bodybuilders' understandings are prioritised . . . viewing drug use from the point of view of the drug user [aims to] show the meaning drug use has in [the drug users] lives' (p. 4). For Shilling and Bunsell (2009), in studying the female bodybuilder as a gender outlaw, the purpose of their research was to 'facilitate a rich portrait of the values, practices, norms and, above all, the lived experiences of the female bodybuilders' (p. 145). Similarly, talking about the aims of their study of physical activity, sport and mental health, Carless and Douglas (2010a) comment:

> Our interest here is less to do with answering the question *What effect does sport/physical activity have on mental illness?* And more to do with exploring the question *What does sport/physical activity mean for you in the context of your life?* To answer this question it is necessary to take seriously the stories individuals tell about their experiences because these stories reveal how they make sense of their lives (in relation to the past, present and future) and the place they give to physical activity and sport across their lives.
>
> (Carless & Douglas, 2010a)

To understand the meanings that people construct, researchers need to understand the particular *contexts* in which they act, and the influence that this context has on thoughts, beliefs and actions. Therefore, qualitative researchers, adopt an *ideographic* rather than a *nomothetic* approach. They typically study a relatively small number of individuals or situations and try to preserve the individuality of these in their analyses, rather than collecting data from large samples and aggregating the data across individuals or situations. The ideographic approach is used to better understand how events, actions and meanings are shaped by the unique circumstances in which they occur.

A major concern and strength of qualitative research is its ability to illuminate the dynamics of *process*. A commitment to studying social life in process, as it unfolds, is a key feature of qualitative research. Here, researchers extend their analyses of the qualities of the social to the ways its processes both enter into, and reflexively constitute, everyday life.

> The social world is viewed as fluid and elastic, so attention is directed to the working definitions and procedures by which the world is given meaning. Seeing people as active agents of their affairs, qualitative inquiry has traditionally focused on how purposeful actors participate in, construct, deeply experience, or imagine their lives.
>
> (Gubrium & Holstein, 1997: 12)

The ability of qualitative research to get at the processes that lead to various outcomes is a major strength of this approach and is something that experimental and survey research is often poor at identifying.

Natural settings, 'being there' and extensive interaction

Bergson (1903/1961) stated that, 'Philosophers agree in making a deep distinction between two ways of knowing a thing. The first implies going all around it, the second entering into it' (p. 1). We can certainly know much about the world by describing it from the outside. However, as Charmaz (2004) reminds us, to understand what living in this world *means*, we need to learn from the inside. Starting from the inside is the initial step to develop a rich qualitative analysis because if we want to gain a deep understanding of any life, we have to enter into it. Charmaz suggests that developing an 'intimate familiarity with the phenomenon means gaining a level of knowledge and understanding that penetrates the experience. Learn the rhythms of actions within it and the design of daily life' (p. 984).

Given their desire to explore the meanings that people attach to their experiences, qualitative researchers prefer to engage with people in their 'natural' settings or environments. Of course, just what is 'natural' is open to debate. For example, how 'natural' is an interview situation about experiences in the gym as opposed to a free flowing conversation that actually takes place in the gym about the same experiences? Putting this issue to one side, it remains that qualitative researchers favour *naturalism* in their research methods. For Avis (2005), methodological naturalism holds that research techniques should be 'familiar to people being studied, respect their beliefs, have similarities with normal social interaction, and leave people undisturbed as far as is possible' (p. 6). Extracting people from their environments where they feel comfortable and placing them in highly structured or manipulated social settings like the formal experiment are, therefore, avoided.

Interviews of various kinds are often arranged at a time and place chosen by the participants so that they feel comfortable and secure in their environment. Likewise, observation sessions are arranged where the participants actually work, perform, or go about their daily lives. Indeed, for qualitative researchers who opt for an ethnographic approach (see Chapter 2), they might decide to participate as a full member of the group to 'immerse' themselves in the phenomenon under study and begin to understand it from the 'inside'. This displays what Gubrium and Holstein (1997) call a commitment to *close scrutiny* and involves the researcher placing themselves in *direct contact* with, or in *immediate proximity* to, the lived world of those being studied in order to understand and document the organisation of social life as it is practiced and experienced. For them:

> While methods of close scrutiny vary, the goals are basically the same: to see the unseen in its own right, to represent the unknown in living colour . . . Qualitative researchers maintain that only close scrutiny can give voice to the eloquence of the commonplace.
>
> (p. 11)

An example of this commitment to close scrutiny, direct contact with, and immediate proximity to, can be found in the two year ethnography of the female bodybuilder as gender outlaw by Shilling and Bunsell (2009) in which Bunsell, herself a qualified personal trainer and regular gym user, 'immersed herself in the routines of this lifestyle by training, dieting and interacting with female bodybuilders' (p. 144). In her study that explored what appearance-focused messages were conveyed by instructors in aerobic classes for women, D'Abundo (2009) utilised both semi-structured interviews and adopted the role of 'participant as observer' who joined in the activities with other class members. Likewise, Spencer (2011) spent four years of participant observation as a fully involved member of a mixed martial arts (MMA) club training and fighting on a regular basis. This carnal experience that involved pain, injury and getting a sense of the rhythms of combat, was supplemented by in-depth interviews with amateur and professional MMA fighters to reveal how in this activity the cultural scripts of masculinity in popular culture are transgressed in various ways.

As indicated above, qualitative research relies on *extensive interaction* with the people being studied. This is because, as Avis (2005) notes, given the desire to explore the meanings that people attach to their experiences, or to view the social world through the eyes of the partici-pants in the research, it is necessary for the researcher to interact with them 'over an extended period and in a fairly unconstrained manner' (p. 5). This leads qualitative researchers, on occasions, to choose open and often unstructured interactions with people going about their daily activities. Of course, this raises the issue of how much time is 'correct' for any given study. In this regard, Wolcott (1994) warns that fieldwork as opposed to *just* being in the field is very different and time alone does not guarantee the breadth, depth, or accuracy of one's information. For him, 'mere presence guarantees rather little' (p. 78). The approach adopted by the researcher and what they do in and with their time in the field is the crucial point.

Adopting a reflexive stance

In qualitative research it is not only the subjective experiences of the par-ticipants in the study that are important but also the *subjectivity of the researcher*. This includes how they themselves affect the ways in which the research is conducted and the findings are interpreted. The connec-tions between the self and study are often powerful forces in shaping many aspects of the research process, from the topic selection to the way data are reported and how these are interpreted. Key aspects of the self that shape all this include gender, age, ethnicity, sexual identity, (dis)ability, religion and social class as well as theoretical orientations and previous experiences. Given this appreciation of researcher *subjectivity*, Finlay and Gough (2003) note how in recent years the notion of *reflexivity* has exploded into academic consciousness as a means by which qualitative researchers can transform the 'problem' of subjectivity (in the eyes of some) into an opportunity.

> The etymological root of the word 'reflexive' means 'to bend back upon oneself'. In research terms this can be translated as thoughtful, self-aware analysis of the intersubjective dynamics between researcher and researched. Reflexivity requires critical self-reflection of the ways in which researchers' social background, assumptions, positioning and behaviour impact on the research process. It demands acknowledgement of how researchers (co)construct their research findings.
>
> (Finlay & Gough, 2003: ix)

Beyond such definitions, numerous forms of reflexivity exist in practice. Finlay and Gough (2003) note the following broad trends: reflexivity as introspection; reflexivity as intersubjective reflection; reflexivity as mutual collaboration; reflexivity as social critique; and reflexivity as ironic deconstruction. Taking these in combination, they argue that reflexivity as a whole has the potential to be a valuable resource for qualitative researchers in helping them to:

- examine the impact of the position, perspective and presence of the researcher.
- promote rich insight through examining personal responses and interpersonal dynamics.
- open up unconscious motivations and implicit biases in the researcher's approach.
- empower others by opening up a more radical consciousness.
- evaluate the research process, method and outcomes.
- enable public scrutiny of the integrity of the research through offering a methodological log of research decisions. (Finlay & Gough, 2003: 16–17)

Vannini, Waskul and Gottschalk (2012) speak of reflexivity as somatic work. Reflexivity for them is the activity of turning back on oneself, or the action of taking the role of the other in examining oneself. Reflexivity can involve putting ourselves in somebody else's shoes and imagining how this other perceives us (see also Smith, 2008). In the context of qualitative research it can also mean examining our assumptions, rapport with participants, choice of topic, research questions, methods, paradigmatic choices, analytical strategies and writing styles.

20

It means coming to terms with how and why the research we do is. . . . 'so us!' It also means examining how our biography shapes what we know and want to know. For example, our gender, age, ethnicity, subcultural identity, class, and religion of residence shape what we know, how we think and feel, and how we are embodied. Being reflexive also means being able to take into account the presence we establish in the field through our (always embodied) methods. In sum, reflexivity means seriously taking into consideration the researcher as a mindful body; a body that is obviously and inevitable present in the research process.

(Vannini et al., 2012: 78)

Day (2012) also notes various forms of reflexivity and how a consideration of each can enhance the thinking, doing and evaluation of qualitative research. Besides *positional* reflexivity that involves considering how the subjectivity and role of the researcher shapes the process of knowledge production, Day makes the case that different forms of reflexivity are required to engage with the multidimensional power dynamics embedded in qualitative research. This involves, for example, considering the power shifts that take place in interviews along with the emotional labour involved. It also involves being aware of the ways in which our research participants are variously located within relationships of power *outside* of the immediate interviewing context, as well as the ways in which we as researchers are also positioned in different power relations that are connected to broader social structures, which can include our location within particular theoretical traditions and approaches.

Of course, as Etherington (2004) points out, adopting a reflexive stance throughout a study is no easy task. She proposes that keeping a *reflexive research journal* or *diary* can help researchers focus on their internal responses to being a researcher and enable them to capture their changing and developing understanding of method and content. In addition, such journals can be used to assist us in reflecting on our roles, 'on the impact of the research upon our personal and professional lives, on our relationships with participants, on our perception of the impact we may be having on *their* lives and on our negative and/or positive feelings about what is happening during the research process' (p. 127). She also suggests that keeping a reflexive research journal can 'help us attend to our senses – what we see, hear, and sense in our bodies – all of which are needed for reflexive monitoring' (p. 128).

This monitoring through a reflexive journal is important because researchers undertaking qualitative often focus on sensitive topics (e.g. career terminating injuries or illness in sport). Therefore, they need to be able to make an assessment of the impact of the research on both the participants *and* themselves (see Chapter 8). For example, in an ethnographic study by Brewer and Sparkes (2011) of how young people experienced parental death and the role of physical activity in the process of coping with this event, Brewer utilised a field diary as a resource for monitoring her emotional and physical status during the course of the study and how this shaped her decision-making, selection and interpretation of events. Likewise, Sparkes and Smith (2012a) adopt a reflexive stance towards their own study of men who have experienced spinal cord injury through sport by examining the possible ways in which their own bodies as researchers shaped, both consciously and unconsciously, their narrative analysis of the participants' lives. This kind of methodological reflexivity is also evident in the 'confessional' tales that researchers provide about their experiences in the field which are examined in Chapter 6.

Prioritise textual data, purposeful sampling and naturalistic generalisations

Qualitative researchers can, and do use numerical data. However, in their attempts to understand the meanings of human action they *prioritise* obtaining and analysing textual data. That is, they generate and analyse nonnumeric data in the form of words, images, sounds and other senses as opposed to attending in any sustained way to quantitative data that is numeric in form. According to Avis (2005), the importance of textual data is that it allows people to express their thoughts and beliefs and explain their actions and events in their own words and on their own terms. He continues:

> This not to say that measurement or relevant information is not of interest to qualitative researchers. A commitment to narrative detail does not imply that qualitative data cannot or should not be summarised in quantitative form, but there is a responsibility to analyse and present textual data in a way that preserves their narrative and social character. This commitment is often demonstrated in qualitative researchers' use of direct quotations to illustrate their findings.
>
> (Avis, 2005: 5)

22

As Krane and Baird (2005) point out, depending on the context of the study, researchers may examine documents written for a group (e.g. athlete handbook), about a group (e.g. newspaper or magazine articles), or by a group (e.g. journals or scrapbooks). These may include formal texts (e.g. published or official documents) or informal texts (e.g. participant journals or diaries). To this must be added photographs, autobiographies, drawings, film, digital forms of data, and web based sources, such as blogs and chatrooms (see Chapter 4).

Examples of the range of textual data, beyond that generated in interviews, used in SEH research is evident in the work of the following. Apostolis and Giles (2011) examined the contents within the *Golf Digest* for 2008 to reveal the ways in which, despite the increase in women columnists and content concerning women in articles or advertisements, the magazine mainly reproduced dominant images about white, wealthy, heterosexual sportswomen. Weber and Barker-Ruchti (2012) considered how female gymnasts' performances of the 1970s were visualised by examining a sample of professional sports photographs and how these constructed and established gender and body standards through their visual construction of gendered and de-gendered gymnastics performances. Likewise, Anderson and Kian (2012) provide a media analysis of the reporting of Aaron Rogers' self-withdrawal (after hitting his head) from an important National Football league game and show how this offers a challenge to the self-sacrifice component of sporting masculinity and the warrior narrative. In contrast, Smith and Stewart (2012) explore the social constructions, body perceptions and health experiences of serious recreational and competitive bodybuilders and powerlifters by drawing on data generated from a discussion forum appearing within an online community dedicated to muscular development.

Others have used published sporting autobiographies as the focus of their analysis. For example, Sparkes (2004) used the autobiography of Lance Armstrong as a resource to explore the changing nature of body–self relationships over time by this sportsman, how these were framed by particular narrative forms, and how the story as constructed by Armstrong acted as a powerful narrative map for other athletes who experience serious illness. Overman (2008) analysed male sporting autobiographies to examine issues such as sex and sexuality, sport and race, the athlete and his body and retiring from sport. Burke and Sparkes (2009) focused on how cognitive dissonance is experienced in one sporting subculture by analysing the published autobiographies of six high altitude climbers.

Finally, Stewart, Smith and Sparkes (2011) investigated the role of metaphor in shaping the illness experience of athletes in twelve sporting autobiographies.

Clearly, the term 'textual data' is wide ranging and opens up endless possibilities for qualitative researchers to select from. It could be argued that depending on the philosophical assumptions, research questions and the purposes of the study that everything and anything can potentially be classed as data. This inclusive definition, of course, raises its own problems in terms of making appropriate selections from what is available in the field. This brings to the fore the central issue of sampling in qualitative research.

The issue of sampling is dealt with in greater detail in Chapter 3. Suffice to say here that various forms of sampling are available to the qualitative researcher that fall under the general term of *purposeful sampling*. This is very different to the kinds of sampling utilised in quantitative studies because qualitative researchers choose an individual, a number of individuals, or a group with whom they have an interest and who they feel will provide 'information rich' cases. Sampling decisions not only include people but also involve sampling of events and concepts, time, processes and place.

Importantly, in qualitative research, N = 1 is permissible and frequently necessary to achieve the depth of understanding required (see Chapters 2 and 3). For example, Gaskin, Andersen and Morris (2010) explore the meanings of sport and physical activity in the life of a 30-year-old man with cerebral palsy. Potrac and Jones (2009) focus on one coach to illuminate the micropolitical strategies that he used in an attempt to persuade the players, the assistant coach and the chairman at his football club to 'buy into' his coaching program and methods. Likewise, Smith and Sparkes (2008b) explore the chaos narrative of one former rugby player who has suffered a spinal cord injury in this sport and the difficulties he encountered in reconstructing his life post-injury.

When working with such small numbers statistical generalisations are not possible or desirable. Indeed, as Maxwell (1996) points out, the value of a qualitative study may depend on its *lack* of external generalisability, in the sense of it being representative of a larger population; 'it may provide an account of a setting or population that is illuminating as an extreme case or ideal type' (p. 97). The notion of generalisability takes on a different meaning for qualitative researchers who speak of such things

24

as naturalistic generalisations, transferability and generativity, all of which are considered in detail in Chapter 7.

Inductive and deductive reasoning

According to Hagger and Chatzisarantis (2011), quantitative researchers engage in very little inductive, 'theory generating' or 'theory building' research – that is truly 'inductive' research. For them,

> much of the development of theory in quantitative psychology applied to sport and exercise arises though the support and con-firmation or lack of support and rejection of research or experi-mental hypotheses through a series of carefully developed cor-relational and experimental studies.
>
> (p. 273)

In contrast, most qualitative research begins with inductive strategies in relation to a set of issues or foreshadowed problems.

Inductive reasoning, according to Angrosino (2007) and Holloway (1997), means going from the specific to the general. The researcher starts with an observation or study of a number of individual cases or incidents and then establishes generalities that link them to each other. Often qualita-tive researchers attempt to 'bracket' their theoretical assumptions prior to collecting data and then see what emerges from the data in their analy-sis. This is a 'bottom up' approach that is concerned with producing descriptions and explanations of particular phenomena, or with devel-oping theories rather than testing existing hypotheses.

For example, during their analysis of the narrative construction of body–self relationships following spinal cord injury in sport, Smith and Sparkes (2005) noticed that the participants often used the term 'hope' in their talk but defined this in very different ways depending upon the narrative type that framed their experiences. Importantly, Smith and Sparkes did not begin their study with a hypothesis about hope. Rather, this important theme emerged from the analysis of their interview data in an inductive manner, as did several other theoretical themes associated with the participants' use of metaphors (Smith & Sparkes, 2004) time tenses (Sparkes & Smith, 2003), and their memories of pain (Sparkes & Smith, 2008a).

This is not to say that qualitative researchers do not use deductive reasoning in their studies. As theories, working propositions and hypotheses begin to emerge, they might move into a more deductive mode that involves the researcher shifting from the general to the specific. Here, researchers start with a general theory from which a conclusion is deducted. They then search for empirical evidence by testing a working hypothesis, a theory, or examining a research question through collecting data from observation and then analysing them. For example, McCarthy and Jones (2007), given their established knowledge of the sports-enjoyment literature, utilised what they call *concurrent inductive and deductive content analysis* in their study of the enjoyment and non-enjoyment among young children in the sampling years of sports participation. In relation to the interview material, deductive analysis was used to identify specific units associated with previous sources of sport enjoyment, while an inductive content analysis was used to generate raw data themes not specifically accounted for by previous research on sport enjoyment and non-enjoyment. Likewise, given that their study was driven by a specific model of resilience that framed their conceptualisation of this phenomenon and shaped the formulation of the research and the interview questions, Galli and Vealey (2008) began by using deductive reasoning. However, their work became more inductive at the point of data analysis, as they searched for concepts, relationships and processes not necessarily accounted for in the original model, but that emerged from the interviews with athletes.

In contrast, Kerr and Males' (2010) study of the motivational experiences and psychological responses of members of an under-performing national lacrosse team at a world championship tournament was deductive throughout as it used predetermined themes and categories from reversal theory to guide the analysis of interview data provided by participants. Finally, with regard to their analysis of data generated in a case study of an elite athlete's use of imagery during rehabilitation from injury, Hare, Evans and Callow (2008) comment as follows:

> The interview guide, which was based on an extensive review of the research literature, provided a deductive analytical framework. Thereafter, analysis of the interview data involved moving back and forth between deductive and inductive approaches . . . this movement allowed for both the verification of deductively driven hypotheses and the exploration of inductive findings that emerge from the multiple interviews.
>
> (p. 411)

Qualitative researchers might, therefore, prioritise inductive reasoning at the start of their study and continue in this vein throughout. Alternatively, they might decide to integrate deductive reasoning as the study progresses, especially if working propositions are developed. They can decide, as in the study by Ryba, Haapanen, Mosek and Ng (2012) on the acute cultural adaption (ACA) of elite female swimmers, to include a mix of inductive and deductive reasoning throughout the study. This mixing is known as *abductive* reasoning. Ryba and colleagues described this process as follows:

> The analytic procedure involved a succession of inductive and deductive processes, which may be described as abductive. Abductive reasoning involves a dialectical movement between everyday meanings and theoretical explanations, acknowledging the creative process of interpretation when applying a theoretical framework to participants' experiences . . . Such a procedure was followed because the aims of the study were to understand what processes constituted ACA for the swimmers (inductive) and to establish whether the swimmers' experiences could be understood through the SDT-based psychological needs (deductive).
>
> (p. 85)

Given the strategies described above, as Schwandt (1997) notes, there is something of a half-truth in the claim that qualitative studies are inductive. For him, qualitative analysis often does indeed begin with the data of specific cases. But then it often (but not always) moves to construct working hypotheses by playing around with ideas and hunches about the data rather than derive those hypotheses in the first instance from established theory. Therefore, as Schwandt suggests, analysis in qualitative research typically involves all forms of inference, including induction, deduction and abduction. For him, 'The claim that qualitative studies are 'inductive' may actually be a way of saying that they reject the hypo-deductive methods of explanation in the social sciences' (p. 70).

Tolerance for complexity and flexible research designs

For Gubrium and Holstein (1997), given that everyday life is not straightforwardly knowable or describable, then, qualitative researchers have to *tolerate complexity* and resist the impulse to gloss over troublesome uncertainties, anomalies, irregularities, and inconsistencies in the interest of 'comprehensive, totalising, or finalising explanations . . . As matter of principle, qualitative inquiry accommodates and pursues the problematic finding or the unanticipated occurrence' (p.13). Given the complexity of the field, and given the search for meanings as these emerge in context as part of an interacting and dynamic process between people and events, then qualitative researchers require *flexible* designs to their studies.

As Hammell (2007) states in her discussion of the contribution of different approaches to understanding quality of life (QOL) after spinal cord injury (SCI), quantitative research is hypothesis driven and requires that researchers predetermine the variables to be measured and thus to identify in advance those factors that they feel are relevant and important to the issue under investigation. For her, this 'inevitably limits the range of possible findings' (p. 124). For example, if 'pain' is not included as a variable in a quantitative study of QOL then pain will not be found to influence QOL. Hammell also notes the inherent problems with attempts to quantitatively measure QOL among people with SCI. In view of this, she supports exploratory forms of inquiry and approaches to understanding an issue as complex as QOL. This is especially so when seeking to understand the QOL perceived by those whose lives may differ from the researchers' by virtue of such factors as, for example, gender, class, race, ethnicity, sexual orientation, age, religion and (dis)ability. As such, she advocates flexible qualitative approaches that can explore both the meaning of QOL for people with SCI and the factors they identify as contributing to the experience of quality in their lives.

Talking of the inherent flexibility of qualitative research, Pitney and Parker (2009) note that researchers often find it difficult to predict the people they will need to interview, the documents they will need to examine, or where and for how long they will need to conduct their observations in the field. Wolcott (1999) summarises this nicely in the following conversation between two ethnographers.

First ethnographer:	Where are you going to do your fieldwork?
Second ethnographer:	I don't know yet.
First ethnographer:	What are you going to study?
Second ethnographer:	That depends on where I go.

(p. 19)

Qualitative researchers usually employ a plan of inquiry that *emerges* or evolves as the research study progresses. As a consequence, they rarely have a rigidly predefined protocol for sampling, data collection and analysis. Instead, Avis (2005) notes, 'they will start with a broad research question and, after negotiating access to people who have relevant experiences to offer, they go on to develop their plan for sampling, data generation and analysis as the study progresses' (p. 5). Due to this flexible and emergent design, qualitative researchers can be sensitive to unanticipated factors or puzzling features that arise in the field and can alter their design as required in relation to the original research question. As Holloway (1997) comments:

> Although researchers draw up an outline of boundaries, they develop and adjust design during the process of the research, and they will decide on particular processes throughout the study. For instance, early assumptions might be wrong. During the course of the research, participants follow different directions from those envisaged initially. When this happens researchers might wish to modify their research design.
>
> (Holloway, 1997: 138)

The need for a flexible and emergent research design is particularly important given that, often in qualitative research, data collection and analysis proceed *iteratively*. This means collecting data and analysing it occurs simultaneously rather than sequentially as in quantitative research. For example, during an in-depth interview the respondent might raise an issue that the researcher had not even thought about at the start of the study which could lead to changes being made in the research design in terms of, the kinds of questions asked during interviewing and the characteristics of the people selected for interview. Likewise, participant observations in the field might alert the researcher to emerging phenomena that require attention which had not been built into the original research design.

Reflecting on their study of expertise in cricket batting, Weissensteiner, Abernethy and Farrow (2009) emphasise that they chose a qualitative approach because their study was largely exploratory in nature and

> required a methodology that was highly generative, had an inherent freedom to explore situation dynamics and the interrelationships of critical components, and was sufficiently flexible to

permit continual redirection of the focus of the inquiry to areas of emerging importance.

(p. 278)

Speaking as *quantitative* researchers Eklund *et al.* (2011) openly acknowledge that from their perspective one of the strengths of qualitative research lies in the flexibility of the investigative process.

Qualitative projects can fruitfully evolve as a function of the data acquisition process in ways that might undermine the integrity of data obtained in traditional quantitative designs. More specifically, qualitative data are often strengthened, rather than compromised (or turned into 'pilot data' as can occur in quantitative studies), by mid-process investigative modifications in response to constraints and investigative challenges. This evolutionary flexibility can produce interesting leads, complexities and alternatives. It can also be particularly useful in applied field settings wherein vantage points for sport psychology research are constantly being re-negotiated with participants and gatekeepers. That is, qualitative researchers can work around situational constraints and changes in available affordances while still obtaining detailed, useful information to address a given research question. This can sometimes keep qualitative studies alive and valid under conditions which might render a quantitative study essentially unsalvageable.

(p. 287)

Grappling with the meanings in qualitative research poses thorny problems and uncertainties. Our attempts to understand the subjective worlds of others can often leave us confused and uncertain. Acknowledging that we do not have the right answers and may not have the right questions allows us to open ourselves to ambiguity. For Charmaz (2004), qualitative researchers need to embrace ambiguity, contradiction and their sense of bewilderment, treating these as signs that they are entering the phenomenon and gaining a deeper understanding of its complexities and processes. Once again, this form of embracing requires a flexible and emergent research design to allow researchers to utilise ambiguity, contradiction and bewilderment as dynamic resources that informs their study as it develops over time.

SUMMARY

In this chapter we have highlighted the problems of defining precisely what qualitative research is given that is it an umbrella term that encompasses a number of research traditions within it. Having acknowledged this issue of difference we suggested that one way to get a flavour of qualitative research is to reflect on some similarities that link together those who choose to conduct inquiry of this nature. One approach to this involved inspecting the philosophical assumptions that inform qualitative research and frame its practice in action. The second approach we suggested involved examining the key characteristics of what qualitative researchers seem to do when they conduct their inquiries.

Throughout this chapter and throughout the book you will note that we have not claimed that qualitative research is inherently better than quantitative research. Rather, we have emphasised that in many ways these are very different. On this issue, Horn (2011) comments as follows.

> I have become resigned to believe that quantitative and qualitative scholars do tread two different roads. However, once we (or at least some of us) realise that we are generally headed in the same direction (knowledge generation and dispersal) and that there is great value in each of our approaches, then we and our students can benefit significantly from each other's work. But, it is important, particularly in our work with students, that we do not deliberately try to discredit the work carried on by those on the 'other road' just so that we can justify our own methodological approach and thus our own survival in a climate of economic meltdown.
>
> (Horn, 2011: 299)

To assist us illustrate and explain some of these differences we have necessarily drawn on ideal types. In so doing, we are acutely aware of the problems associated with such a strategy. As Sparkes (1992) notes, this strategy only reveals the central tendencies and dimensions of any given paradigm and inevitably glosses over certain distinctions within a paradigm and does not give full weight to internal disagreements about procedures and perspectives. Furthermore, as Silverman (2000) points out, our strategy can potentially set up highly dangerous dichotomies or polarities.

For him, 'At best, they [paradigms] are pedagogic devices for students to obtain a first grip on a difficult field: they help them to learn the jargon. At worst, they are excuses for not thinking, which assemble groups of sociologists into "armed camps", unwilling to learn from each other' (p. 11). In a similar fashion, Weed (2009a) in considering the problems associated with paradigmatic behaviours, recognises that it is all too easy to frame debates about difference in terms of 'us' and 'them'. This can have a number of negative consequences.

First, Weed (2009a) suggests that if debates are conducted solely for the purposes of fully converting 'them' (the 'other') to 'our' point of view, then the debate will not be able to benefit from any consideration of the 'others' critique for one's own position. A second consequence noted by Weed is as follows:

> [R]ather than engagement in a genuine argument, paradigmatic behaviour can reduce debates to mere contradiction of the position of the 'other', with the dismissal of 'their' position being justified on the basis that is derived from an incommensurable paradigm. The implications of such paradigmatic behaviours are that they diminish the quality of debate surrounding difficult issues around the nature of knowledge and science as applied to sport research, and ultimately adversely affect the quality of knowledge that sport research generates.
>
> (Weed, 2009a: 312)

Against this backdrop, we have tried to use ideal types for the best of purposes. That is, as pedagogic and heuristic devices to enable students and established scholars to access a complex area with a view to making informed and principled decisions about how they might proceed as qualitative researchers, if indeed, they wish to proceed at all. We have no desire to convert anybody to qualitative research. Equally, we have no intention of using labels to construct a negative 'other' with a view demeaning alternative positions in favour of ours. Rather, we wish to celebrate difference and acknowledge the complexities involved in all forms of research in the field of SEH.

CHAPTER 2

TRADITIONS IN QUALITATIVE RESEARCH

In Chapter 1 we proposed that qualitative research was a camp that contained a number of communities and traditions. In this chapter we seek to give a brief overview of some of these and give a flavour of how each tradition has been used within research in sport, exercise and health (SEH). These traditions are not presented in any order of importance. We do not wish to infer that one is better than the others. Rather, we note the differences and the value of each in exploring issues of interest in SEH.

ETHNOGRAPHY

The term ethnography derives from the Greek *ethnos* (meaning 'people'), and *graph* (meaning 'writing'). Various theoretical orientations and models of practice inform the work of ethnographers. There are, however, a number of shared commitments. Most importantly, this includes a commitment to the first-hand experience and exploration of a particular social or cultural setting on the basis of (though not exclusively by) participant observation. Angrosino (2007) notes a number of basic principles and features that link ethnographers.

- A search for patterns proceeds from careful observations of lived behavior and from detailed interviews with people in the community under study. When ethnographers speak about 'culture' or 'society' or 'community', it is important to keep in mind that they are speaking in terms that are generalised abstractions based on numerous bits of data in ways that make sense to the ethnographer who has a global overview of the world or cultural whole that people living in it may lack.
- Ethnographers must pay careful attention to the process of field research. Attention must always be paid to the ways in which one gains entry to the field site, establishes rapport with the people living there, and comes to be a participating member of the group. (Angrosino, 2007: 14)

Angrosino (2007) goes on to define ethnography as the 'art and science of describing a human group – its institutions, interpersonal behaviors, material productions, and beliefs' (p. 14). In support of this definition O'Reilly (2012) offers the following:

> Ethnography is a practice that evolves in design as the study progresses; involves direct and sustained contact with human beings, in the context of their daily lives, over a prolonged period of time; draws on a family of methods, usually including participant observation and conversation; respects the complexity of the social world; and therefore tells rich, sensitive and credible stories.
>
> (O'Reilly, 2012: 3)

The key characteristic of *cultural interpretation* is embedded in many of the definitions of ethnography offered in the literature. As Krane and Baird (2005) note, the aim of ethnography is to understand the culture of a particular group from the perspective of the group members. It is, therefore, the group culture that provides the insights into the behaviours, values, emotions and mental states of group members and so ethnographers employ multiple methods to gain a comprehensive understanding of the social environment and perceptions of the members of the social group. In order to make such cultural interpretations Atkinson (2012) suggests that ethnographers seek to generate theory through experiential education. That is, seeing, doing and feeling first-hand is deemed to be the best way to believing, knowing and theorising sociologically about members of another culture.

> Although a contested argument, a realist ethnographer might only 'truly' know a culture after one perceives him/herself to be a practicing member of said culture. When one achieves roles, statuses and identities in the culture; views themselves as a member of the culture and shares a commitment to the reproduction of the culture, ethnographic modes of knowing are shifted into high gear.
>
> (Atkinson, 2012: 32–33)

Ethnography necessarily involves both a *process* for accomplishing cultural interpretation (for example, doing fieldwork), and also the presentation itself, that is, the *product* of the research which ordinarily takes its form in prose (for example, to present an ethnography of something).

34

Although ethnographers utilise a range of data gathering techniques, it is the use of *participant observation* that is most distinctive about this tradition (see Chapter 4). This is based on the key assumption that by entering into a close and relatively prolonged interaction with people in their everyday lives, ethnographers can better understand the beliefs, motivations and behaviours of those involved than they can using any other approach. For Atkinson (2012) this is a process of knowing a subject by doing and becoming through what he calls *immersed observation*. As Sparkes (2009a) and Sparkes and Smith (2012b) emphasise, this immersion develops embodied ways of knowing through an engagement with all of the senses as fieldwork is conducted.

The participant observer role can taken on many forms ranging along a continuum from complete or 'pure' observer to complete or 'pure' participant, and these forms may change during the course of a study depending on the circumstances (see Chapters 3 and 4). For Atkinson (2012), the notion of participant observation captures the dual role of the ethnographer in that 'one is both a participant in the culture, but at the same time is an academic observer' (p. 27). Negotiating these roles, gaining access to various groups and developing trust in the field can be problematic and will be discussed in more detail in later chapters.

In terms of the product, ethnographers produce rich descriptions of the culture or subculture studied. For Wolcott (2010) ethnography's most important contribution is in purposeful and thorough description. For him, this is what ethnographers do and that is how they continue to develop the ethnographic potential. He states:

> Don't be cowed by the idea that we only describe – our contribution comes as well out of what we assess as being worthy of our descriptive effort. If description is something you do well, consider that a gift. If you are not good at it, work to enhance your capabilities.
>
> (p. 141)

Increasingly, researchers in SEH are utilising ethnographic approaches in their studies. Recent examples include the following: the structures of 'jock' culture, its spatial dynamics and forms of embodiment (Sparkes & Partington, 2007; Sparkes, Partington & Brown, 2010); Parkour as an emerging urban 'anarcho-environmental' movement (Atkinson, 2009); women's varied bodily experiences in exercise and sport (D'Abundo,

2009); cognitive dissonance in mountain climbing (Burke, Sparkes & Allen-Collinson, 2008); the embodied dynamics of martial arts as a religion (Brown, Jennings & Sparkes, 2010); the construction of alternative femininities via gender manoeuvring in women's roller derby (Finley, 2010); the moral worlds and experiences of embodiment among middle-class cage-fighters (Abramson & Modzelewski, 2011); the carnal experience of mixed martial arts fighting and how it transgresses the cultural scripts of masculinity in popular culture (Spencer, 2011); the snowboarding body as historical, gendered, cultural, sensual, affective and political (Thorpe, 2011); the subculture of rock climbing and how 'informal' rules get defined in this self-governed sport (Bogardus, 2012); the organisational functioning of a national sport organisation (Wagstaff, Fletcher & Hanton 2012); embodied forms of knowing and learning in yoga (Atkinson, 2012); and the unwritten and unsaid rules of boxing as a field and how this shapes the gendered dynamics of the gym and the experiences of those within in it (Paradis, 2012).

These ethnographies illustrate the amount of time researchers devote to being in the field and also indicate the different positioning they might have at the start of the study in terms of being an 'insider' or an 'outsider' in the group. For example, in their two-year ethnographic study of the multiple meanings of sport and exercise in a high security prison (Martos-Garcia, Devis-Devis & Sparkes, 2009), the researcher in the field (Martos) was not a member of the prison community and had to spend a great deal of time dealing with gatekeepers in the form of government agencies before he could gain access to a suitable prison in Spain. Equally, as an outsider he had to devote a great deal of time once inside the prison to developing trusting relationships with the prisoners, the prison guards and the prison administrators.

Long-term immersion is also evident in McGrath and Chananie-Hill's (2009) two-year ethnographic study of normalising gender transgression through bodybuilding. Here, however, McGrath herself had been participating in amateur bodybuilding competitions for two and a half years, and been weightlifting for a total of four years. Her status, as an 'insider' in the bodybuilding subculture gave her access to the 'backstage' behaviours normally inaccessible to 'outsiders'. McGrath's involvement in bodybuilding competitions allowed her to develop close bonds of trust and mutual understanding with interviewees which puts them at greater ease when discussing their own perceptions and experiences.

McGrath and Chananie-Hill's (2009) work illustrates the benefits of being an insider or a member of the group you wish to study in terms of gaining access and developing rapport. Insider status can, like familiarity, breed analytical contempt, however, in that much may be taken for granted and the researcher may find it difficult to 'make the familiar strange' in the research setting. Often, it is easier for the naive outsider to raise questions and problematise the mundane and taken-for-granted nature of everyday activities and beliefs. Such issues will be discussed in greater detail in Chapters 3 and 4 where we reflect on the choices that need to be made prior to conducting an ethnographic study.

PHENOMENOLOGY

Phenomenology, derived from the Greek 'phainomenon', is the study of phenomena (appearances), things as they present themselves to, and are perceived in, human consciousness. For Allen-Collinson (2009) phenomenology is a complex, multifaceted, mutable, nuanced and contested philosophy that defies simple characterisation because it does not have a single unified standpoint. In her review, she considers the following interlinking strands within the phenomenological movement: constitutive/transcendental, hermeneutic, and existential phenomenology. Not surprisingly, Norlyk and Harder (2010) argue that adopting a phenomenological approach to research is challenging because of the difficulties of firstly understanding a complex philosophy and then deciding how to accomplish this by putting it into practice in a phenomenological study. They identify at least eighteen schools of phenomenology, and note that even though there are some commonalities between them, there are also some distinct differences in terms of their purposes and forms of data analysis.

One thing phenomenologists do have in common, however, is their rejection of scientific realism and the accompanying view that the empirical sciences have a privileged position in identifying and explaining features of a mind-dependent world (see Chapter 1).

> Phenomenologists insist on careful description of ordinary conscious experience of everyday life (the *life-world*), a description of 'things' (the essential structures of consciousness) as one experiences them. These 'things' we experience include perception (hearing, seeing, and so on), believing, remembering,

deciding, feeling, judging, evaluating, all experiences of bodily action, and so forth. Phenomenological descriptions of such things are possible only by turning from things to their meaning, from what is to the nature of what is.

(Schwandt, 1997: 114)

To produce such descriptions, phenomenologists engage in a process of *reduction* or *epoché*. This entails the suspension of everyday taken-for-granted assumptions about a phenomenon, or at least attempts to identify these explicitly and set them aside, in order to suspend or *bracket* the *natural attitude*. The purpose of this is to allow the researcher to be fully present to the instance of the phenomenon being described by the participant so that she or he can arrive at and describe the essential characteristics of the phenomenon. The goal of phenomenological reduction is to distil the phenomenon down to its core meaning or *essence*. This is done by a process called *free imaginative variation*. Here, the researcher searches for the most invariant meanings of the phenomenon, or the fundamental meanings that are essential for the phenomenon to present itself as it is. In this process of free imaginative variation, as described by Berry, Kowalski, Ferguson and McHugh (2010), 'one changes the parts of the phenomenon to see if the phenomenon still remains identifiable. In doing so, the researcher becomes aware of those features that cannot be removed or changed in order for the phenomenon to exist' (p. 297).

Phenomenology is a philosophy and an attitude to human existence rather than a specific research method or set of prescribed techniques or procedures. It is difficult to describe how this approach is put into action. Allen-Collinson (2009) notes that there have been numerous and varied efforts at operationalising phenomenology as a specific empirical approach. One of these is provided in the following guidelines for undertaking this kind of research by Giorgi (1985).

(1) The collection of concrete, 'naïve' descriptions from participants', as co-researchers.
(2) The researcher's adoption of the phenomenological attitude.
(3) An impressionistic reading of each description to gain a feel of the whole.
(4) The in-depth re-reading of the description to identify 'meaning units', which capture specific aspects of the whole.
(5) Identifying and making explicit the psychological significance of each meaning unit.

38

(6) The production of a general description of the structure(s) of the experience with the aim of letting 'the phenomena speak for themselves'.

(Giorgi, 1985: 151)

In relation to SEH, Kerry and Amour (2000) signalled the promise and potential of phenomenological research approaches. More recently, others, such as Allen-Collinson (2009), Hockey and Allen-Collinson (2007), and contributors to a special edition of *Sport, Ethics and Philosophy* (2011, Volume 5) entitled 'An introduction to the phenomenological study of sport', have endorsed such claims and provide some initial steps towards outlining not only the promises of phenomenology for the study of SEH, but also what such an undertaking might entail.

The influence of phenomenology in research into SEH is evident in the growing numbers of studies that use this approach. The following are some examples. Drawing directly on the work of Giorgi (1985), Berry *et al.* (2010) adopt what they describe as an empirical phenomenological approach to explore young adult women exercisers' body self-compassion. Scott-Dixon (2008) uses the same approach to investigate the experiences of larger female athletes in strength and power-based sports to better understand how they negotiate their identities as athletes and women, and how they navigate 'fitness' and 'fatness'. In contrast, Clegg and Butryn (2012) draw on existential phenomenology to explore the embodied experiences of practitioners of parkour and freerunning. For them, this kind of phenomenology provides a unique framework for examining human experience in the world,

focusing on the tension and 'interpenetration' between one's body, life experiences and meaning . . . existential phenomenology is a research method that focuses on identifying a particular experience, giving a rich and full account of it and incorporating it into a life-text.

(p. 322)

Crust, Keegan, Piggott and Swann (2011) also use existential phenomenology to investigate the experiences of long distance walkers. In a similar fashion, Allen-Collinson and Hockey (2011) analyse the sensory dimensions of the lived sporting body via the haptic (that is, sense of touch) experience of middle/long distance running and scuba diving.

Ravn and Ploug Hansen (2013) make use of this form of phenomenology to deal with how sensory experiences can be described and analysed in movement activities such as dance. In contrast, Bidonde, Goodwin and Drinkwater (2009) adopt a hermeneutic phenomenological stance to study older women's experiences of a fitness program. Likewise, Burke and Sabiston (2010) utilise this stance to examine breast cancer survivors' experiences of subjective well-being in relation to their participation in a climb on Mt. Kilimanjaro.

In recent years, stimulated by the work of Smith, Jarman and Osborn (1999), and Smith and Osborn (2003), a form of phenomenology known as *Interpretive Phenomenological Analysis* (IPA) has become increasingly popular within psychology and the social sciences. For Smith, Flowers and Larkin (2009), IPA is concerned with 'understanding personal lived experience and thus with exploring person's relatedness to, or involvement in, a particular event or process (phenomenon)' (p. 40). This involves a commitment to exploring, describing, interpreting and situating the means by which participants make sense of their experiences.

The influence of IPA within SEH is evident in the work produced by a growing number of scholars. Recent examples have focused on the following topics: athlete experiences of disordered eating in sport (Papathomas & Lavallee, 2010); understanding exercise adherence and dropout from gym users (Pridgeon & Grogan, 2012); the personal experiences of wheelchair rugby coaches in the development of their athletes who had entered their sport after acquiring a spinal cord injury (Tawse, Bloom, Sabiston & Reid, 2012); the experiences associated with burnout in elite soccer coaches (Lundkvist, Gustafsson, Hjalm & Hassmen, 2012); experiences of fear and anxiety in extreme sports (Brymer & Schweitzer, 2012); and the experiences of adversity and perceptions of growth following adversity in elite female athletes (Tamminen, Holt & Neely, 2013).

The emergence of IPA within the social sciences in general has not gone without critique (for example, Chamberlain, 2011). Likewise, in SEH Allen-Collinson (2009) has raised a number of concerns about its use when viewed from the more phenomenological, 'open' and participant-focused end of the phenomenological spectrum. For example, the oft-cited rationale for employing phenomenology in IPA-based studies is that it enables the exploration of participants' subjectivity, experiences and perceptions. As Allen-Collinson however points out:

40

As these are by no means specific to phenomenology but a general goal of much qualitative research in general, the rationale is fundamentally blunted and it is left to the reader to speculate as to why a phenomenological perspective in particular was chosen.

(p. 288)

Further problems Allen-Collinson (2009) identifies relate to the phenomenological–interpretational balance in some IPA research, the over reliance on semi-structured interviews as the primary method to gather data, and the use of various forms of thematic content analysis in IPA studies to examine the participants' understandings of a phenomenon. This said, Allen-Collinson does not deny the usefulness of IPA-based studies, some of which, as she says, are excellent, perceptive and phenomenologically acute. Rather, her intention is 'to raise awareness of some of the problems that *may* occur when studies depart radically from a phenomenological grounding and ethos, or are not explicit about how and why they employ phenomenology specifically, as opposed to other qualitative studies' (p. 288). The use of IPA in SEH continues to be a source of debate and we reflect on this further in Chapter 5.

GROUNDED THEORY

The notion of grounded theory was initiated by the work of Glaser and Strauss (1967) and their book *The Discovery of Grounded Theory* in which they called for a systematic, yet flexible, approach to analysing qualitative data. Since then, as Bluff (2005) argues, this tradition has developed in many directions and resulted in various 'camps' of grounded theorists who differ in what they think the term means and how to go about operationalising research. One of the most influential and articulate advocates of grounded theory is Charmaz (2005, 2006) who adopts a constructivist perspective on this topic which adheres to the central characteristics and assumptions of qualitative research as outlined in Chapter 1.

According to Charmaz (2006: 2), grounded theory can be described as 'a systematic, yet flexible methodology for collecting and analysing qualitative data to construct theories that are grounded in the data themselves'. For her, the term 'grounded theory' refers to both a *method* of inquiry and to the *product* of inquiry. She notes, however, that researchers commonly use the term to mean a specific mode of *analysis* that leads to the development of inductive middle-range theories.

> A major strength of grounded theory methods is that they provide tools for analysing processes . . . A grounded theory approach encourages researchers to remain close to their studied worlds and to develop an integrated set of theoretical concepts from their empirical materials that not only synthesize and interpret them but also show processual relationships.
>
> (Charmaz, 2005: 507–508)

Given their aim to generate theory *from* data, rather than just impose theory *on* data, grounded theorists seek a theoretical sensitivity which allows them to develop insight and an awareness of relevant and significant ideas while simultaneously collecting and analysing data on a given topic of interest throughout the research study (Bluff, 2005; Holloway, 1997). The early analysis of data helps the researcher focus on further data collection and engage in theoretical sampling that is guided by ideas that have significance for the emerging theory. In turn, these data are used to refine the emerging analysis until a point of theoretical saturation is reached. Whereas *data saturation* refers to the point at which the information collected, transcribed and analysed begins to repeat itself (that is nothing new is being found), *theoretical saturation* is about the selection of cases that are most likely to produce the relevant data that will discriminate or test emerging theories. Consequently, as Charmaz (2005) points out, grounded theory entails an inductive–deductive approach that develops abstract ideas about participants' meanings, actions and worlds, and, most importantly, seeks specific data to fill out, refine and check the emerging conceptual categories. For her, the end result is 'an analytic interpretation of the participants' worlds and of the processes constituting how these worlds are constructed' (p. 508).

Grounded theory has had a strong influence on research in SEH. For example, Atkinson (2012) provides a detailed description of how he both conceptualised and used grounded theory in his ethnographic study of Ashtanga Yoga. Other recent grounded theory studies have focused on the following topics: parental involvement in competitive youth sport settings (Holt, Tamminen, Black, Sehn & Wall, 2008); the delivery of video-based performance analysis by youth soccer coaches in England (Groom, Cushion & Nelson, 2011); training adherence in elite school age athletes (Way, Jones & Slater, 2012); successful long-term physical activity behaviour change, grounded in relevant 'real' life experiences (Hutchinson, Johnson & Breckon, 2013); the antecedents, specificity and ceiling effects of golfers' implicit theories of sport ability (Slater, Spray & Smith, 2012); and a better understanding of the psychological factors involved in training and competition in mixed martial arts (Massey, Meyer & Naylor, 2013).

The growth of grounded theory in SEH has not been without its tensions. A lively debate has taken place between Weed (2009b, 2010) and Holt and Tamminen (2010a, 2010b) on the use of grounded theory methodology in sport and exercise psychology research. In his review of papers that claim to be using grounded theory in four leading sport and exercise psychology journals, Weed (2009b) makes the case that most failed to meet even the most basic quality criteria to substantiate this claim. As such, the term 'grounded theory' becomes something of a meaningless label and illustrates that many who think they are conducting research using this approach are not actually doing so. In response, Holt and Tamminen (2010a) criticise elements of the search strategy used by Weed (2009b) and some of the conclusions forwarded, but also reinforce many of the points he makes. They then proceed to suggest six pointers for creating 'optimal conditions' for grounded theory.

Weed's (2010) reaction clarifies points of agreement and provides counterarguments for the criticisms raised. The response by Holt and Tamminen (2010b) then extends the debate by suggesting ways in which researchers can plan grounded theory studies in a manner that demonstrates understanding of research philosophies, methodologies and methods, in relation to their guiding principle of *methodological coherence*. More recently, Hutchinson, Johnson and Breckon (2011) argue in their review of grounded theories in exercise psychology that most studies in this field demonstrate a poor understanding of the grounded theory methodology or fail to present an adequate account of the research process. They recommend that:

> To further legitimise grounded theory as a form of enquiry within exercise psychology and to encourage greater research rigor in all grounded theory applications, it is crucial that both authors and reviewers understand the tenets of this approach and the limitations associated with a number of previous studies.
>
> (p. 247)

LIFE HISTORY AND NARRATIVE

Talking of life-history methodology, Schwandt (1997) makes the following comment:

> Also called the biographical method, this is a generic term for a variety of approaches to qualitative study that focus on the generation, analysis, and presentation of the data of a life history (the unfolding of an individual's experiences over time), life story, personal experience narrative, autobiography, and biography. Data can be generated from interviews as well as personal documents (letters, journals, diaries, and so forth).
>
> (p. 82)

Additional data generating resources mentioned by Plummer (2001) include possessions and 'biographical objects', photographs, videos and films. Web-based resources such as personal blogs, Twitter, Facebook, and so on can also be used by life historians in their quest to understand the personal lives of people within a culture, the norms and values of the culture, and the reasons people give for their beliefs and behaviour (see Chapter 4).

While the terms life history and life story are often used interchangeably, a number of scholars have pointed to important differences between them. Atkinson (1998) defines the life story as follows:

> The life story is the story a person chooses to tell about the life he or she has lived, told as completely and honestly as possible, what is remembered of it, and what the teller wants others to know of it, usually as a result of a guided interview by another . . . A life story is a fairly complete narrating of one's entire experience of life as a whole, highlighting the most important aspects.
>
> (p. 8)

According to Plummer (2001) life stories can be used as both a *resource* and a *topic*. When life stories are used as resources researchers use these to see what insights they may bring to understanding some aspect of social life or the cultural world. In contrast, when life stories are used as topics, researchers see them as matters of investigation in their own right. That is, as topics of interest in themselves. Here, different questions are asked. For

44

example, how does the person come to tell a particular life story in a particular way at a given moment in time? Why and how do they tell it in certain ways and with what consequences?

While accepting such a definition of the life story and recognising its potential as both resource and topic, Hatch and Wisniewski (1995) suggest that 'an analysis of the social, historical, political and economic contexts of a life story by the researcher is what turns life story into a life history' (p. 125). Likewise, Schwandt (1997) notes that life history approaches seek to interrelate the private and the public, the personal and the social. This is done by connecting private, subjective perspectives to meanings, definitions, concepts and practices that are public and social. Therefore, just eliciting the life story of an individual as told during interviews or other means is not enough. To engage in the work of constructing a life history requires that the researcher locate the life story and its events in the history and politics of the time so that the dialectical process between the agency of the individual and the constraints of social structure can be made evident. As Plummer (2001) states:

> More broadly, life history research at its best always brings a focus on historical change, moving between the changing biographical history of the person and the social history of his or her lifespan. Invariably, the gathering of a life history will entail the subject moving to and fro between the developments of their own life cycle and the ways in which external crises and situations (wars, political and religious changes, employment and unemployment situations, economic change, the media and so forth) have impinged on this. A life history cannot be told without a constant reference to historical change, and this central focus on change must be seen as one of life history's great values. Thus life stories can become guides to 'people of their times'.
>
> (Plummer, 2001: 39–40)

A growing number of scholars within SEH have utilised a life history approach. Recent examples have focused on the following topics: the experiences of overtraining and the complex dynamics of this phenomenon at the individual level (Richardson, Andersen & Morris, 2008); how exercise contributed a sense of meaning, purpose and identity to the life of one runner diagnosed with schizophrenia (Carless, 2008); Master and Veteran elite runners' senses of embodiment as ageing social actors

(Tulle, 2008); the experiences of a young women left disabled by an accident and her journey to becoming a British Paralympic wheelchair tennis player (Kavanagh, 2012); the dynamics of pride and shame of an elite bodybuilder as his body became smaller following a career ending injury (Sparkes, Batey & Owen, 2012); and the experiences of an elite athlete of living with and eventually dying from cancer (Sparkes, Perez-Samaniego & Smith, 2012).

Of course, life historians are not the only group of qualitative researchers that draw on life stories as both a resource and a topic. Narrative researchers, in particular, focus on the stories told by people about their experiences and use these for a number of analytical purposes (Gubrium & Holstein, 2009; Riessman, 2008). While there is no one singular definition of what narrative research is, a common thread is the assumption that our lives are storied and that the self is narratively constructed. According to Medved and Brockmeier (2004), autobiographical stories are self-narratives by which we give situation-specific answers to the questions: 'Who am I?' and 'What is my life about?' For them, in telling such stories, 'people give meaning to their experiences within the flow and continuously changing contexts of life . . . All this is done not only in narratives about the past and the present, but also about future times and places' (p. 747). Narratives provide a structure for our very sense of selfhood and identity. Therefore, as we tell stories about our lives to ourselves and to others so we create a narrative identity.

Gubrium and Holstein (2009) claim that stories are actively composed with people artfully picking and choosing from what is experientially available to articulate their inner lives. Importantly, in strategically constructing their accounts, people simultaneously organise their experience in the process. Besides being composed, stories are also staged, and performed for particular effects and purposes that can include the claiming of specific narrative identities. With these points in mind, Smith and Sparkes (2009a) offer the following core characteristics of narrative inquiry:

- Meaning is basic to being human and being human entails actively construing meaning.
- Meaning is created through narrative, and is a storied effort and achievement.
- We are relational beings, and narratives and meanings are achieved within relationships.
- Narratives are both personal and social.

46

- Selves and identities are constituted through narratives, with people relationally doing and performing their storied selves and narrative identities.
- Being human is to live in and through time, and narrative is a primary way of organising our experience of temporality.
- The body is a storyteller, and narratives are embodied.

Given these characteristics, Woike (2008) comments, 'Narrative analysis may be a particularly good choice for researchers interested in complex, subjective experiences, as well as intentions, patterns of reasoning, and attempts to find meaning in personal experiences' (p. 434). Consequently, Riessman (2008) suggests, narrative researchers are interested in the *practices of storytelling* (the narrative impulse – a universal way of knowing and communicating), the *collection of narrative data* (the empirical materials, or objects of scrutiny), and *narrative analysis* (the systematic study of narrative data – which can take many forms) (see Chapter 5).

Importantly, the stories that people tell can be interrogated for *what* they tell us about the individual, the group, or the phenomenon. Equally, these same stories can be analysed in terms of *how* they are told and *performed* by individual and groups in certain sets of circumstance and for certain purposes in order to construct the self and any given phenomenon in different ways (see Chapter 5). As Gubrium and Holstein (1998) point out, on one side of narrative analysis we may focus 'on *how* a story is being told', whilst on the other side, we may have a 'concern for the various *whats* that are involved—for example, the substance, structure, or plot of the story' (p. 165). This dual focus, they suggest, is one feature that distinguishes narrative research from many other forms of qualitative work. The analysis of narratives and biography, therefore, adds a new dimension to qualitative research by focusing not just on what people say and the things and the events they describe but on how they say it, why they say it and what they feel and experienced. In this process, connections are made between the individual teller of the story and the structural aspects of the telling in terms of how this is shaped by the resources provided by and the demands of the host culture and society.

Within the domain of SEH, Smith (2010), and Smith and Sparkes (2009a, 2009b, 2012) have pointed to the analytical strengths and benefits that narrative inquiry can provide. These include the following:

- To reveal the temporal, emotional and contextual quality of lives and relationships.
- To honour much of the complexities of life as lived.
- To instigate personal and social change.
- To connect with bodies and generate a strong sense of the lived, fleshy body.
- To illuminate the subjective worlds of individuals and groups.
- To appreciate a person as a unique individual with agency *and* as someone who is socially situated and culturally fashioned, thereby telling us much about a person or group as well as society and culture.

Scholars in SEH have utilised various forms of narrative inquiry to explore a range of phenomena. Topics focused on include the following: the gendered nature of the flow narratives and experience in a whitewater canoeing club (Sparkes & Partington, 2003); narrative mapping of the body in different sporting contexts and its influence on how young athletes perceive self-ageing (Phoenix & Sparkes, 2006, 2007, 2008); the mid-life nuances, negotiations, and construction of identities in sport and physical activity (Partington, Partington, Fishwick & Allin, 2005); how men with severe mental illness re-story their lives through sport and exercise (Carless & Douglas, 2008a, 2010); how men who have suffered SCI and become disabled through sport reconstruct their lives (Smith, 2013a, b; Smith & Sparkes, 2004, 2005, 2008a, 2011; Sparkes & Smith, 2002, 2005, 2008a, 2011); the complete initiation or hazing experiences of former athletes into male sports teams in the USA (Waldon, Lynn & Krane, 2011); ageing and the different ways a group of mature bodybuilders resist a narrative of decline (Phoenix & Smith, 2011); and how fighters interpret their bodily injuries, how this impacts on their masculine identities, and how injury affects their conformance to the normative masculinity of mixed martial arts (Spencer, 2012).

Of course, narrative inquiry does not have to rely on data elicited during interviews and can analyse storylines and their effect in other contexts (see Chapters 1 and 4). For example, Boyle, Millington and Vertinsky (2006) analyse the narratives of gender, race and disability that are interwoven in the film *Million Dollar Baby*. Similarly, McKay and Roderick, (2010) examine the conflicting narratives infused with prolympism and nationalism in the media reporting of the collapse of Australian rower Sally Robbins in the 2004 Olympics Games. Pike (2011) analyses policy documents, reports and media articles to tease out the various meanings inherent in the Active Aging Agenda and the manner in which they problematise older people as part of a wider moral panic. Likewise, McGannon and Spence (2012) interrogate the construction of exercise narratives within a women's health section of a Midwestern US newspaper in order to reveal the taken-for-granted assumptions and prevailing meanings about women's exercise and health and their implications for self and subjectivity.

Given that narrative research is informed by a number of theoretical approaches it is not surprising to learn that tensions exist between them. Smith and Sparkes (2006) identify several tensions relating to the ontological status of narrative and being a storyteller or story analyst. In addition, Smith and Sparkes (2008b) review a range of contrasting perspectives within narrative studies regarding how selves and identities are understood to be constructed over time that adopt a 'thick individual' and 'thin social relational' view at one end of a continuum and a 'thin individual' and 'thick social relational' view at the other end. Similarly, Sparkes and Smith (2008b) examine the different assumptions that inform the work of scholars operating within the traditions of narrative constructivism and narrative constructionism. The differences and tensions between these perspectives feed into how various forms of narrative analyses are conducted in terms of their purposes and outcomes, which will be the subject of our attention in Chapter 5.

CRITICAL OR OPENLY IDEOLOGICAL RESEARCH

The term 'critical' can have many meanings within qualitative research. In some ways it might be better to speak of openly 'ideologically orientated inquiry' that would include traditions influenced by different kinds of critical theory, such as, neo-Marxism, feminism, Freireism, queer theory, lesbian, gay, bisexual and transgender (LGBT) studies, critical race theory, postcolonial studies, critical disability studies, crip theory, action research and other participatory forms of inquiry. These traditions inform a critical social science that according to Schwandt (1997) aims to integrate theory and practice in such a way that 'individuals and groups become aware of the contradictions and distortions in their belief systems and social practices and are then inspired to change those beliefs and practices' (p. 24). For him, this critical social science is also practical and normative and not merely descriptive. It rejects the possibility of a disinterested social scientist and is orientated toward social and individual transformation. Schwandt further notes that this critical approach is foregrounded on a critique of instrumental, technical reasoning as this kind of thinking actually aims to eliminate crises, conflict and critique. In contrast, critical inquiry supports a kind of reasoning that is practical, moral, and ethically and politically informed.

While there are a number of critical theories that inform the critical approach, a core idea is that knowledge is structured by existing sets of social relations. The aim of a critical methodology is to provide knowledge which engages the prevailing social structures as these are seen by critical researchers, in one way or another, as oppressive in nature. One of the central intentions of critical inquiry is *emancipation*. That is, enabling people to gain the knowledge and power to be in control of their own life. The language and intent of this approach is overtly political, and seeks to dig beneath the surface of historically specific, oppressive, social structures to focus on moments of domination, ideology, hegemony and emancipation in social life with a view to instigating both individual and social change.

While critical inquiry is sympathetic to qualitative forms of research that take reality to be constructed and sustained through the meanings and actions of individuals, it sees some weaknesses in this approach. For critical researchers, achieving a correct understanding of individuals' meanings is a necessary preliminary to social inquiry but is not the whole substance of the theoretical enterprise. They argue that focusing only on the subjective meanings of action tends to imply that social reality is nothing over and above the way people perceive themselves and their situation. For them, however, social reality is not simply structured by concepts and ideas but is also structured and shaped by historical forces and economic and material conditions. These things also structure and affect the perceptions and ideas of individuals so that 'reality' may be misperceived as a consequence of the operation of various ideological processes. Uncovering these processes and explaining how they can condition and constrain interpretations of reality are vital requirements that are largely neglected by various other forms of qualitative research.

Critical researchers see much qualitative research as suffering from 'macro blindness' in that it tends to ignore the unequal power relationships within which people operate when their realities are constructed in terms of social class, gender, sexual orientation, (dis)ability, race, ethnicity and religion, and so tells us little about how individual and group

50

behaviour is influenced by the way that society is organised. Thus, the central line of tension between critical, participatory, action-orientated researchers, and other forms of critical inquiry, is in the call to action, whether this is in terms of internal (individual) transformation or external social transformation.

Against this backdrop researchers in SEH have utilised a critical form of inquiry known as participatory action research (PAR) that is committed to change and seeks to actively involve participants in the research process and product. Thus, PAR is self-consciously collaborative and centres on working *with* rather than *for* participants and communities. Examples of PAR within SEH include the following. Blodgett, Schinke, Smith, Peltier and Pheasant (2011) conducted PAR with Aboriginal community members on promoting physical activity in their own cultural contexts with a view to addressing issues of social injustice through locally-developed efforts that were grounded in trust, relationship-building, co-learning, empowerment, mutual benefit, and long-term commitment as well as a rebalancing of power relations amongst the community and academic co-researchers. Similarly, Dupuis *et al.* (2012) developed an innovative PAR project that brought together persons living with dementia, family members, recreation professionals from a range of settings, Alzheimer Society staff and researchers who worked together to consider the notion of leisure and its meanings for persons living with dementia.

Within the domain of SEH, those whose work is informed by feminism and poststructuralist have made major contributions to the field, particularly with regard to the understanding of power dynamics. As Hargreaves and Vertinsky (2007) note regarding contributions to their edited book entitled *Physical Culture, Power and the Body*:

> The different chapters cover different historical periods and social contexts, but a key feature of them all is the relation between the personal and the social body. This is fundamentally a relation of power linked to other key people, ethnicities, genders, histories, ideologies, religions, institutions, and politics . . . It is clear that the body in question is socially constructed – influenced, changed, adapted, reproduced according to social relations and social structures – and that integral to these processes are unequal relations of power.
>
> (Hargreaves & Vertinsky, 2007: 2)

Likewise, Bolin and Granskog's (2003) edited volume called *Athletic Intruders* investigates women's place in sport and exercise from a socio-cultural vantage point provided by the fields of anthropology of sport, sociology of sport, and feminism. The collection illustrates that women's participation in sport and exercise has not come without struggle into the sports areas marked by male hegemony, such as, bodybuilding and motorcycle riding. Each chapter addresses women's somatic experiences and their consequences for the transformation of women's lives as well as the cultural context in which they are located. More recently, these themes have been continued via the studies of, for example, McGrath and Chananie-Hill (2009), and Shilling and Bunsell (2009) on the nature of gender transgression through bodybuilding, and Scott-Dixon's (2008) study of the experiences of larger female athletes in strength and power-based sports and how they negotiate their identities as athletes and women, and navigate 'fitness' and 'fatness'.

In terms of poststructuralist thinking within SEH the work of Michel Foucault on the power/knowledge/self nexus has been highly influential. Markula and Pringle (2006) provide a detailed introduction to the key ideas of Foucault (for example, discourse, disciplinary power, panopticism, biopower, technologies of the self, and governmentality), and why these are useful for studying SEH. They then illustrate these ideas in action by drawing on a range of examples of how Foucault's work has been used within sports studies as well as using their own research into sport, fitness and physical activity in contemporary culture. For example, in the section of the book that examines Foucauldian interpretations of the body and lived experiences in sport and exercise, Markula and Pringle explore a number of key issues that include the discursive construction of physically active bodies and the healthy body; the connections between health, fitness and the ideal body; how bodies are trained and subsequently disciplined in sport and physical activity settings; and how people actively resist becoming 'docile' bodies.

The core concepts discussed by Markula and Pringle (2006) run through the work of others working from a Foucauldian perspective in SEH. For example, Thorpe (2008, 2011) looks at how technologies of the self and the media messages shape discourses of femininity within snowboarding cultures. Foucault's notion of disciplinary power is used by Scott (2010) to explore the discursive construction, regulation and performance of the body in the context of the swimming pool. Lang (2010) illuminates how surveillance and conformity operate in competitive youth swimming to produce docile, submissive and disciplined bodies, while Johnson and Russell (2012) highlight similar processes at work in terms of how elite athletes construct their gendered body in competitive swimming. A study of the body practices of swimmers by McMahon, Penney and Dinan-Thompson (2012) also draws on concepts from Foucault, such as disciplinary power, surveillance, classification and regulation to inform their analysis. In contrast, Hanold (2010) uses a Foucauldian framework to show how the ultra-running body becomes a desired body beyond the marathon and how these same desires produce multiple and complex subjectivities for female ultra-runners.

Various forms of poststructural thinking also inform the work of those using queer theory in SEH. In her overview of queer feminist cultural studies theories and methodologies, Fusco (2012) argues that 'There is no quintessential queer methodology . . . Instead, all interrogations and interpretations start from a critique of the (hetero)normative discourses and practices of gender and sexuality that take place at the expense of non-normative experiences' (p. 152). Such a position is evident in the contributions to *Sport, Sexualities and Queer/Theory* edited by Caudwell (2006). Focusing on a range of queer bodies, as well as heterosexual experiences, the volume illustrates how the use of queer theory can document complex subjectivities and expand our knowledge of sexuality with a view to challenging sexual prejudice in sport and the relations of power that aid its production. For Sykes (2006),

> Queering sport studies has the potential to alter how we think about sexualities, desires and bodies . . . Queer theorising moves across interdisciplinary boundaries, employs deconstructive logics of paradox and contradiction while self-reflexively assessing it unpredictable yet necessary political and ethical dimensions.
>
> (pp. 26–27)

With regard to queering the domain of sport psychology, Krane, Walson, Kauer and Semerjian (2010) note that queer theory can be effectively used to destabilise heteronormativity while recognising the existence of lesbian, gay, bisexual and transgender (LGBT) identities in sport by confronting dominant practices that privilege heterosexuality and establish alternative practices and structures that value all sexual and gender identities. Developing this theme, Kauer and Krane (2012) use a transnational, queer feminist analysis to explore the intersections of sexuality, gender, race, social class and nation, and examine how these combine to perpetuate heterosexism and homonegativism in women's sport. They highlight the confluence of multiple axes of oppression, and reveal the contradictions of lived experiences with binary categorisations of gender and sexual orientation. Kauer and Krane conclude that, 'there is a continued imperative to critique heteronormative, homonormative, and international representations of LBTs in sport as well as the treatment of all women in sport' (p. 10).

Calling for a rethinking of subjectivity in sport and exercise psychology, McGannon and Busanich (2010) acknowledge the contribution that research grounded in feminist cultural studies has made to understanding the complex relationship between socio-cultural influences, the self, and women's physical activity participation in sport and exercise psychology. Having advocated that more work be done in sport and exercise psychology using this approach, they then signal some problems. These include the tendency of feminist cultural studies to adhere to a neoliberal view of the self, and the ways in which they conceptualise power dynamics within hegemonic relationships as they impact on understandings of the self in the contexts of body management practices. Accordingly, McGannon and Busanich suggest that a feminist poststructuralist perspective can make a major contribution as a theoretical tool 'to expand a feminist understanding of sociocultural influences on the self and women's physical activity in light of its differential view of power, ideology, and the self' (p. 216). Similarly, using women boxers as an example, Caudwell (2011, 2012) considers the ways that sports feminists theorise the complex power relationships of gender and sexuality in sport. She explores the usefulness of adopting the (traditional) feminist historical model and feminist waves of theory (first wave, second wave and third wave) and cautions against the implicit assumption of a logic of progression in these and also the suppositions made by many so-called third wavers.

CASE STUDY

Case studies are commonly used in qualitative research and also by quantitative researchers. The case study is not a methodological choice but a choice of what is to be studied. That is, by whatever methods used, we

54

choose to study *the case* of something. As Stake (2005) points out, a case study is both a *process* of inquiry about the case and the *product* of that inquiry. That is, 'I am doing a case study of a chosen phenomenon and I will present my findings in the form of a case study'.

According to Schwandt (1997) the terms 'case' and 'unit of analysis' are often used interchangeably in social research. He notes, however, that for the qualitative inquirer, the term 'case' means something more than just 'N'. For him, a case is typically regarded as a 'specific and bounded (in time and place) instance of a phenomenon selected for study. The phenomenon of interest may be a person, process, event, group, organisation, and so on' (p. 12). Instead of seeking answers to such questions as 'how much' or 'how many', case study research is useful for answering 'how' and 'why' questions.

> A case study is expected to catch the complexity of a single case. A single leaf, even a single toothpick, has unique complexities – but rarely will we care enough to submit it to case study. We study a case when it is of very special interest. We look for the detail of the interaction with its contexts. Case study is the study of the particularity and complexity of a single case, coming to understand its activities within important circumstances . . . The case is one among others. In any given study, we will concentrate on the one. The time we spend concentrating on the one may be a day or a year, but while we so concentrate we are engaged in case study.
>
> (Stake, 1995: 1–2)

As Stake (2005) points out, however, not everything is a case. A child may be a case, easy to specify. Likewise, a doctor may be a case, but *his or her doctoring* probably lacks the specificity, the *boundedness* to be called a case. For him, if we are moved to study it, the case is almost certainly going to be a functioning body, that is, a specific, unique and 'bounded system'. Certain features will be recognised as being within the system, that is, within the boundaries of the case, while other features will fall outside of it. As researchers, therefore, we can ask: 'What is this a case of and what questions do we wish to ask of it?'

Stake (2005) identifies three kinds of case study: the intrinsic, the instrumental and the collective case study. An *intrinsic* case study is undertaken because the researcher wants a better understanding of this particular case. Here, the study is not undertaken primarily because the case represents other cases or because it illustrates a particular trait or problem. Rather, it is studied because in all its particularity and ordinariness, this case is itself of interest:

> [T]he purpose is not to come to understand some abstract construct or generic phenomenon . . . [T]he purpose is not theory building – though at other times the researcher may do just that. The study is undertaken because of an intrinsic interest in, for example, this particular child, clinic, conference, or curriculum.
>
> (p. 445)

In contrast, Stake (2005) states that an *instrumental* case study is where a particular case is examined mainly to provide insight into an issue or to redraw a generalisation:

> The case is of secondary interest, it plays a supportive role, and it facilitates our understanding of something else. The case is still looked at in depth, its contexts scrutinised and its ordinary activities detailed, but all because this helps to pursue the external interest. The case may be seen as typical of other cases or not. Here the choice of case is made to advance understanding of that other interest. We simultaneously have several interests, particular and general.
>
> (Stake, 2005: 445)

As Stake (2005) is quick to point out there are no hard-and-fast lines distinguishing intrinsic case study from instrumental, but rather a zone of combined or overlapping purposes. Against this, when there is even less interest in one particular case, a number of cases may be studied jointly in order to investigate a phenomenon, population, or general condition. Stake classifies this as the *multiple* case study or *collective* case study. Here, the instrumental case study is extended to several cases that are chosen because it is believed that investigating these will lead to a better understanding, and perhaps better theorising, about a still larger collection of cases.

Given the nature of case study as described the selection of cases for study becomes of crucial importance. As Stake (2005) emphasises, 'Achieving the greatest understanding of the critical phenomena depends on choosing the case well . . . My choice would be to choose that case from which

56

we feel we can learn the most' (pp. 450–451). This might mean studying the case that is most accessible to us or the one we can spend the most time with. In terms of purposeful sampling strategies the following have been suggested as useful for guiding the selection process: extreme or deviant cases; particularly typical cases; maximum variation cases that are as different as possible from each other; critical cases; and convenience or opportunistic cases that just happen to become available to the researcher (for a discussion of sampling see Chapter 3).

A number of qualitative researchers in SEH have offered various reasons why we might use a case study. For example, Giges and Van Raalte (2012), in their editorial to a special edition of *The Sport Psychologist* (Volume 26, Number 4) on the use of case studies in this field suggest that this approach can provide valuable insights into the influence, appropriateness and effectiveness of performance intervention and enhancement techniques or strategies as well as allowing the athlete to reflect on and describe his or her performance behaviours and outcomes. For them, 'Case studies can allow for in-depth exploration of a variety of situations and issues. They can include unexpected occurrences, unique and innovative interventions, unusual circumstances, or typical experiences that illustrate important principles in consultation' (p. 483).

Not surprisingly, the case study approach is popular within SEH. For example, Singer and Cunningham (2012) draw directly on the work of Stake (2005) in their case study of the diversity culture of an American university athletic department. This study represented one specific case from a larger, ongoing body of work related to diversity best practices of athletic departments that are member institutions of the National College Athletic Association (NCAA).

> The university and athletic department that was the focus of this study was one of the few recipients of an award that is given to athletics departments that exemplify excellence in diversity. In efforts to understand the intricacies of how diversity is managed in this particular athletic department, we employed an *intrinsic case study* approach (Stake, 2005). We were interested in the unique attributes of this particular university and its athletic department, and in illuminating the stories of those 'living the case' (Stake, 2005) or intimately involved in the operations and functioning of this organisation.
>
> (Singer & Cunningham, 2012: 653)

Others examples of case study work in SEH include the following that focus on sporting injuries: the experiential dynamics of career termination and transition for a professional (McKenna & Thomas, 2007); the rehabilitation experience of a professional rugby player following anterior cruciate ligament reconstructive surgery (Carson & Polman, 2008); the function and outcome of using imagery during rehabilitation from injury for an Olympic athlete (Hare *et al.*, 2008); how perceptions of pain are influenced by changing settings and the behaviours of others during the period from initial injury to stabilisation (Heil, 2012); and vicarious trauma in sports coaches and the difficulties they faced having witnessed a serious athletic injury (Day, Bond & Smith, 2013).

Other experiences focused on by case study work include the following: how a 70-year-old physically active man uses leisure and health practices to accomplish a positive ageing identity (Phoenix & Sparkes, 2009); the meanings of sport and physical activity in the life of a man with cerebral palsy (Gaskin *et al.*, 2010); the perceived usefulness and benefits of using a personal motivation video for a professional mountain bike racer (Tracey, 2011); the progression from a cognitive–behavioural, psychological skills training approach with a rugby football player experiencing adjustment and mood disorder to a psychodynamic and interpersonal engagement with the client using themes from Buddhist psychotherapy (Thompson & Andersen, 2012); and 'real life' ethical decision-making in sport psychology that occurred in the context of a symposium on sexual transgressions in sport conducted during a professional conference (Dzikus, Fisher & Hays, 2012).

A number of tensions and misunderstandings are attached to the case study approach. As Flyvbjerg (2006) notes, the standard misunderstanding is that one cannot generalise from a case study of one, and so a single case-study approach cannot contribute to scientific development and understanding. Other misunderstandings about case study research identified by Flyvbjerg, include the following: (a) the case study is most useful for generating hypotheses, whereas other methods are more suitable for hypotheses testing and theory building; (b) the case study contains a bias towards verification; (c) it is often difficult to summarise specific case studies; and (d) theoretical knowledge is more valuable than practical knowledge. In a similar fashion, Day *et al.* (2013) unpack some of the misunderstandings of case study research and highlight various benefits, including the ability of case studies to develop theory-focused generalisations, or what is sometimes called analytical generalisations (see

58

Chapter 6). Regardless of these misunderstandings, as Flyvbjerg (2006) states, 'A scientific discipline without a large number of thoroughly executed case studies is a discipline without systematic production of exemplars, and a discipline without exemplars is an ineffective one' (p. 219).

SUMMARY

In this chapter we have reviewed six key traditions within the domain of qualitative research. In terms of the basic assumptions that inform each (see Chapter 1) there are a number of similarities. This said, as indicated, there are a number of differences, which are often subtle. These differences play themselves out further in the ways that researchers go about collecting and analysing their data, and will be focused upon in Chapters 4 and 5. At this stage, the important thing is to get a flavour of and a feel for the various traditions as part of developing an awareness of the diversity of approaches that are available to qualitative researchers in SEH. You may already find yourself drawn more towards some traditions than others, often without really knowing why. Our intention in the chapters that follow is to enable the reader to develop these early likings for some traditions over others in a critical manner so that by the time they embark on a research project they will be able to make informed and principled decisions about which tradition or traditions are appealing, relevant and useful for them engage with.

CHAPTER 3

GETTING STARTED WITH SOME PRE-STUDY TASKS

Qualitative researchers make many decisions and engage in various study tasks before they actually begin collecting data through field work. The time and effort spent on working through these pre-study tasks and the decisions that emanate from them is not wasted. As Glesne and Peshkin (1992) point out, any research plan will probably change as the field-work progresses and the researcher needs to be flexible to accommodate these changes as required. They emphasise, however, that without any plan, the study may flounder, suffer many false starts, and be needlessly extended. Some of these pre-study tasks and decisions are as follows.

LITERATURE REVIEW

A literature review is both a process (that is, something you do at various stages of the research process) and a product (that is, an identifiable part of your thesis or paper). Regarding the process, Chenail, Cooper and Desir (2010) note that reviewing the literature in qualitative research can be a challenging matter in terms of why, when, where and how we should access third-party sources in our work. Novice researchers can often receive conflicting advice on this issue. Some scholars argue for a literature review while others advocate little or no review of the literature before beginning a qualitative study. These disagreements about when and how to conduct a literature review revolve around the notion of 'bias'.

For Chenail *et al.* (2010), the 'none' or 'little prior literature' group justify their position by noting how the infusion of ideas regarding the phenomenon in question can fill discovery-orientated researchers with potentially biased perspectives. Too much exposure to the literature and too much 'theory', they argue, could prevent researchers seeing and hearing that which might otherwise be observed in the field and in the data collected as well as in the analysis of this data. As Corbin and Strauss (2007: 35) warn, 'the researcher does not want to be so steeped in the literature that he or she is constrained or even stifled by it. It is not unusual for students to become so enamored with a previous study or the theory, either before or during their investigation, that they become literally paralyzed'.

Reflecting on the role of theory within the tradition of ethnography Wolcott (1995) feels that it is 'overrated in terms of what most of us actually accomplish through our research. In theory-driven descriptive accounts, theory is more apt to get in the way than to point the way, to tell rather than to ask what we have seen' (p. 186). He is against the kind of thesis or dissertation construction that contains in the second chapter the 'typically tedious review of the literature' alongside an 'equally tedious recital of "relevant" theory' (p. 187). An alternative approach he offers involves introducing theory into the final account in whatever role is *actually* played during the field research and write-up. Thus, for his students, issues of theory and the review of related literature can often be reserved for the closing chapters of the dissertation, 'where a self-conscious but genuine search for theoretical implications and links *begins* rather than ends' (p. 187). Wolcott concludes as follows: 'A student (or colleague) without a theory is in a far better position to discover (and eventually even appreciate) how theory serves than someone who has been "given" a theory by someone else, no matter how well intended the gift' (p. 188). Such views are typical of those who advocate a 'findings-driven' strategy whereby the emerging results of the study suggest areas of the literature that the researcher might usefully access. In this 'after-the-fact' or 'a posteriori' model, researchers can wait until the analysis is completed before they access the literature, and in their written accounts of this model in action they can present the results of their post-hoc reflective comparison in either the results or discussion sections of their thesis or paper (Chenail *et al.*, 2010).

In contrast, those holding a more traditional position on the literature review argue, like Pitney and Parker (2009), that it serves to provide a context for conducting the proposed study. This is sought by first establishing what is known about a phenomenon within a field of inquiry and then locating the theoretical/conceptual frameworks that have informed, enhanced, or limited our understanding of the phenomenon so that gaps in our knowledge can be identified and questions generated for a new study to explore. Pitney and Parker add that this process also allows the researcher to demonstrate their grasp of a particular topic and their familiarity with related research so that the originality and significance of the proposed study can be assessed. For this 'a priori' group, it is important that researchers situate their work within an ongoing discussion of the topic among peers as this provides some 'beginnings' for the researcher's thinking and may assist clarity without making the final point of their reflections about data a certain matter.

> The critical issue with regard to familiarity with existing literature is not what one knows or believes, but *how one makes use of that knowledge in designing and conducting qualitative research*. The goal is to become familiar with the background literature without becoming tied to or directed by particular theories or models.
>
> (Haverkamp & Young, 2007: 285, emphasis added)

In addition, Corbin and Strauss (2007) argue that the literature review can be used 'to provide questions for initial observations and interviews' and 'to stimulate questions during analysis' (p. 37). The literature can assist researchers in addressing ethics committees of various kinds by providing them with a list of conceptual areas to be explored in the study and examples of how previous researchers on the topic have dealt with key ethical issues (see Chapter 8). Using the literature can also be useful to researchers in others ways, for example helping them consider the kinds of sampling procedures they might want to employ.

Against this backdrop, Chenail *et al.* (2010) recommend that, instead of seeing it as something that is done only in a particular phase of a study, qualitative researchers should utilise research literature in four functional ways *throughout* the research process, to

(a) define the phenomenon in question;
(b) identify the research gap in which the study is situated;
(c) support the methodological choices made in the study; and
(d) compare and contrast what was learned through the results of the study with what was previously known and not known about the phenomenon.

Each of these will now be briefly considered.

Using a literature review to define the phenomenon

The work of relevant others is selectively used by researchers to articulate their area of curiosity and make their initial orientation or posture towards a phenomenon transparent. This helps establish the credibility and relevance of their work and plays an important part in establishing the context and purpose of the study, its rationale, and its anticipated contribution to the field. Chenail *et al.* (2010) emphasise that researchers who adopt a qualitative analytical approach should remember that *evidence is not a matter of quantity*. The sheer number of references cited does not necessarily make for a good literature review. It needs to be *highly selective* and only focus on *relevant* studies and findings. In other words, don't parade how much you've read, but instead use the literature for certain needs and to guide various choices.

Using the literature to identify the research gap

Reviewing the literature the researcher might find that information about the phenomenon seems to be lacking or unknown. Thus, a 'gap in the knowledge' base is identified that needs to be filled. To support this 'non-knowledge' posture, researchers will necessarily need to acknowledge previous work in the area as part of their literature review. This orientation, Chenail *et al.* (2010) suggest, helps researchers build a case for (a) the importance of their research (for example, 'the study has the potential to add to our knowledge of the phenomenon or possibly challenge that which we thought we already knew about it') and (b) the credibility of using a qualitative approach to conduct the study. Both of these points are also useful in assisting the researcher establish the wider significance of their local studies.

Using the literature to support methodological choices

By reviewing the literature to see how others have conducted studies on a given phenomenon, researchers can get ideas about which methodological approach is best suited to their own study. As Chenail *et al.* (2010) note, by using 'research method citations, qualitative researchers can make more transparent the methodological traditions and practices that organized their decision-making in creating the design for their study' (p. 91). They argue that by connecting their methodological choices within established qualitative research traditions, 'researchers can also help guide their reviewers and readers to consider the relevant paradigmatic quality criteria from which to judge the method from both conceptual and operational perspectives' (p. 91). For example, if the researcher cites the work of ethnographers in their methods section of the thesis or paper, they are alerting the reader that they have conceptualised and operationalised their procedures within a specific qualitative tradition (see

Chapter 2), and that the quality criteria appropriate for this tradition should be used to judge the work (see Chapter 7). Not to use such a citation system as part of communicating why they have chosen a certain methodological approach and certain data gathering techniques might open up the researcher to criticism from those who hold to different methodological and paradigmatic assumptions (see Chapter 1).

Using the literature review to discuss results

Normally, at the end of a thesis or a paper, the researcher provides a 'discussion' section (see Chapter 6 on representing findings). Here, they compare and contrast what was learned in their study with what was previously known and not known about a phenomenon and the implications this might have for current policy or practice and future research in the area. As Chenail *et al.* (2010) point out, 'Juxtaposing what was found and not found with what was known and not known in the previous research literature can provide clarification and focus and help researchers and readers of research reports alike make sense of current findings' (p. 92). Using this tactic, researchers can highlight how their findings support or confirm findings from others studies, challenge these, or actually provide something completely new to the knowledge base.

Most papers published in SEH journals provide a literature review of some kind. For example, Sparkes and Partington (2003) begin by using a literature review to examine how the phenomenon of flow had been defined and most importantly, how it had been researched in previous studies. They noted that the majority of research on flow had been quantitative in nature and that little qualitative research had been conducted. Thus, they used the literature to identify a gap that needed to be filled by the inclusion of qualitative work in general. Then, by reviewing the kinds of qualitative research conducted into the flow phenomenon, Sparkes and Partington pointed out that a narrative approach was noticeable by its absence. Having done this, they proceed to making strong case for the use of a narrative approach and use the literature to support this methodological choice and the kinds of questions it asks. Finally, having presented their findings on the ways that flow is narratively constructed within a white water canoeing club they returned to the literature to situate their findings and highlight the potential that narrative approaches have to both add to, and extend, our understanding of the flow phenomenon in sport.

GENERATING QUALITATIVE RESEARCH QUESTIONS

The literature review normally assists the researcher formulate their research questions and the statement of purpose. As Agee (2009) reminds us, 'good questions do not necessarily produce good research, but poorly conceived or constructed questions will likely create problems that affect all subsequent stages of the study' (p. 431). The process of generating and then refining questions are critical in shaping all phases of a qualitative study.

As Willig (2004) points out, most qualitative research studies are guided by one or more research questions, and research questions are not the same as hypotheses. A hypothesis is a claim, derived from existing theory, which can be tested against empirical evidence. It can be either rejected or retained. In contrast, a research question is open-ended and cannot be answered with a simple 'yes' or 'no'. Rather it calls for an answer that provides detailed descriptions and, where possible, explanations of a phenomenon.

> *Qualitative research questions* identify the process, object or identity that the researcher wants to investigate. It points us in the direction without predicting what we may find. Good qualitative questions tend to be process orientated. They ask *how* something happens rather than just *what* happens . . . Qualitative research questions are always provisional because the researcher may find that the very concepts and terminology used in the research question are, in fact, not appropriate or relevant to the participants' experiences . . . Qualitative research is open to the possibility that the research question may have to change during the research process.
>
> (Willig, 2004: 19)

This view is supported by Agee (2009) who notes that qualitative questions focus on the *why* and *how* of human interactions. Questions need to articulate what a researcher wants to know about the intentions and perspectives of those involved in social interactions. Agee also emphasises that in qualitative research the questions will change during the process of the inquiry and that, once in the field, questions may emerge that were not even thought of at the start of the study. For her, 'Good qualitative questions are usually developed or refined in all stages of a reflexive and interactive inquiry journey . . . To extend the journey metaphor, it is helpful to think of research questions as navigational tools that can help a researcher map possible directions but also to inquire about the unexpected' (p. 432).

A good example here is provided by Spencer (2011) who acknowledges that his initial interest in mixed martial arts (MMA) and bodies was based on a number of central research questions, or as he puts it 'puzzles'.

> What are the ways in which bodies are produced to be able to participate in the arduous sport of MMA? Exactly, what goes on 'behind closed doors'? Of equal importance, I believe, what does it take to become and what is the *experience* of *becoming* an MMA practitioner? How do fighters incorporate body techniques into their technical corpus? What does the accumulation of bodies for a common goal bring to the lives of those participating in MMA? How do those participating in the sport of MMA see themselves in terms of their individual identities in relation to other fighters and those outside of the sport of MMA?
>
> (Spencer, 2011: 9)

The following are further examples of those who have gone through a similar process to generate qualitative research questions in SEH.

- How do breast cancer survivors give meaning to their experiences of climbing Mt. Kilimanjaro? (Burke & Sabiston, 2010).
- How and why do women bodybuilders as multiple transgressors get defined as gender outlaws and how does this shape their experiences? (Shilling & Bunsell, 2009).
- How do people learn life skills though their involvement in regular competitive sport programmes? (Holt, Tamminen, Tink & Black, 2009).
- How do young adult women exercisers experience body self-compassion? (Berry *et al.*, 2010).
- How do disability sports coaches learn to coach? (McMaster, Culver & Werthner, 2012).

Having articulated such how, why and what questions, the researcher is in a better position to articulate a *statement of purpose* or *problem statement* for their study. The following are examples of statements of purpose: 'The purpose of this study is to examine the learning experiences of coaches in disability sport' (McMaster *et al.*, 2012); 'The purpose of this phenomenological investigation was to explore the lived, embodied experiences of traceurs' (Clegg & Butryn, 2012: 323); and 'The aim of this qualitative investigation was to explore body image in female swimmers, and to see whether there were differences in accounts between adolescents and adults, thereby addressing the failure of previous research to consider possible maturational differences' (Howells & Grogan, 2012: 101). Given the emergent nature of qualitative inquiry and its research design, early statements of purpose should be seen as tentative and subject to change as the study develops.

DATA GATHERING TECHNIQUES AND ANALYSIS

Having reviewed the literature, generated your research question and provided a statement of purpose, researchers are then in a position to think about the kinds of data they will need to answer their questions. Qualitative researchers have a wide range of data sources and data collection techniques to draw on, including participant observation, interviews (of various kinds), documentary sources, and visual methods (for example, photography, film), to name but a few (see Chapter 4). In choosing what data gathering technique or techniques to use, careful consideration needs to be given to what you want to learn.

> Different questions have different implications for data collection. In considering options, choose techniques that are likely to (1) elicit data needed to gain understanding of the phenomenon in question, (2) contribute different perspectives on the issue, and (3) make effective use of the time available for data collection.
>
> (Glesne & Peshkin, 1992: 24)

The same can be said of how you might begin to analyse your data both while it is being collected and afterwards (see Chapter 5). Thus, if you decide to include interviews in your research project, how might you analyse the data generated? Similarly, if you include photo-elicitation as a data gathering technique, how might you analyse the data generated? Such questions need careful consideration before the study begins and most certainly before any data collection takes place.

Given the flexible nature of qualitative research design this is not to say that different forms of analysis cannot be introduced into a study once data have been collected should it be deemed necessary, and provided there is a coherent rationale for doing so. This choice, however, would be in addition to those that have already been selected prior to the study beginning. Importantly, at this pre-study stage, depending on the data gathering technique or techniques chosen, it is possible to construct a provisional framework in the form of an interview guide or observational schedule (see Chapter 4).

SAMPLING

Sampling involves making informed and strategic choices about which people, places, settings, events, and times are best for gaining the data you need to address your research questions. Given the emergent nature of qualitative research you will make sampling decisions both when you create your proposal and as the study progresses. As Pitney and Parker (2009) comment, 'some findings prompt you to look for confirming data or explore aspects of a phenomenon that you did not anticipate. In these cases, you may need to interview participants whom you did not originally consider' (p. 42).

There are two important sampling issues in qualitative research. The first, according to Schwandt (1997), is *selecting* a field site in which to study some phenomenon (or developing a case through which to study some phenomenon), and *sampling within* this case or field site. For him, the locus of study (that is, where one studies) is not the object of the study (that is, what one studies). The researcher does not study a place or site (school, health club, and so on) but investigates some phenomenon (social process, human action) *within* a place or site. Schwandt points out that the selection of a site such as, a health club (or the definition of a case) is generally not made on the basis of a random sampling procedure designed to yield a representative site. The logic of probability sampling is rarely applied in site selection. Rather, the site, place, or person is chosen on the basis of a combination of criteria including availability, accessibility and theoretical interest.

> A *single* place may be chosen because in that site one has good reason to believe that (1) the human action or social process going on there . . . is critical to understanding, testing, or elaborating

68

on some theory or generalized concept of that social process, or (2) the social process unfolding there is extreme, deviant, or unique, or (3) the site or case is particularly revelatory or previously inaccessible. *Multiple* places, cases, or sites for study are chosen to facilitate comparisons either because they are likely to yield predictable contrasts in understanding the definition of social action or because they are likely to show the same or similar definition of social action.

(Schwandt, 1997: 141)

For example, in his ethnographic study that investigated bodybuilding, drugs and risk, Monaghan (2001) began with a pilot study that surveyed 15 bodybuilding gyms, 12 leisure centres, 3 needle exchanges and a Well Steroid User Clinic in 12 towns located in South Wales. He also undertook participant observation at physique competitions and various other settings (for example night clubs, respondents' homes, and 'gyms' in backstreet garages). Based on this, Monaghan eventually selected commercial bodybuilding gyms as the main ethnographic site, and the main ethnographic study was conducted on a time-sampling basis at four gyms over a sixteen month period. These gyms were identified as 'hard core' by bodybuilders themselves, meaning they had the requisite equipment and atmosphere associated with the serious business of creating the 'perfect body'.

Once the above decisions have been made a second set of sampling considerations become important that involve sampling *within* the place(s), site(s), or case(s). According to Schwandt (1997), to explore the nature and definitions of social action within a particular site, the researcher considers sampling across time, processes, occasions or events, and people. In terms of selecting people, Holloway (1997) suggests that generally between four and forty participants is normal depending on the specific approach being used. In certain circumstances, and for particular purposes, however, more or fewer participants may be required. For example, Carless and Sparkes (2008) provided case study material of three men with severe mental illness and the meanings that physical activity has in their lives. In contrast, Dunn and Holt (2004) interviewed twenty seven male intercollegiate ice hockey players in their investigation of a personal-disclosure mutual-sharing team building activity, while Pickard and Bailey (2009) drew upon data generated by semi-structured interviews with sixty three elite young ballet dancers to explore their crystallising experiences in this activity.

Sampling in qualitative research is best described as *purposive* or *purposeful* in which an attempt is made to gain as much knowledge as possible about the context, the person or other sampling units. Researchers choose an individual, a number of individuals, or a group in whom they have an interest and who they feel will provide 'information rich' cases based on them having specific characteristics. These may be members of a subculture or community who have knowledge of the setting or the phenomenon that is of interest to the researcher. As Holloway (1997) notes, 'This means that sampling is not fixed in advance but is an ongoing process guided by emerging ideas' (p. 142). Silverman (2000) points out that purposeful sampling is often treated as a synonym for *theoretical* sampling which is concerned with constructing a sample which is meaningful theoretically, because it builds in certain characteristics or criteria which help to develop or test a theory or explanation.

Within the general categories of purposeful sampling Patton (1990) describes fifteen subtypes. These include the following:

- *Criterion-based sampling.* The researcher predetermines a set of criteria for selecting places, sites, or cases. Participants are chosen because they have a particular feature, attribute or characteristic, or have a specific experience.
- *Typical case sampling.* Participants are chosen because they fit in with a norm for a given population or reflect the 'average' person, situation, or instance of the phenomenon of interest.
- *Maximum variation sampling.* Researchers define the dimensions of variation in the population that are most relevant to their study and then systematically select individuals, sites, or times that represent the most important possible variations of these dimensions. A range of different perspectives on one situation are explored by recruiting people from a variety of backgrounds. Often attempts are made to find views which are as different as possible to disclose the range of variation and differentiation in the field. This form of sampling assists researchers to explore multiple facets of a problem and investigate issues holistically.
- *Deviant case sampling.* Researchers deliberately seek participants, programmes, or situations that deviate substantially from the norm. They examine situations that are classified as unusual or distinctly 'non-average'. Choosing deviant cases can guard against any tendency to select only cases that support your theory in that these can act as 'negative' instances that challenge the theories that are in use.

70

- *Critical case sampling.* Similar to deviant case sampling, researchers select their samples to deliberately examine cases that are critical for the theories that they began the study with, or that they have subsequently developed. These extreme cases often provide a crucial test of these theories and can illuminate what is going on in a way that representative cases cannot.
- *Snowball (chain, network, nominated) sampling.* Researchers rely on participants to direct them toward others who meet the study's criteria for inclusion. They might begin with a few participants who then identify others 'like them' who they feel would provide information rich cases and be useful for the researcher to meet.
- *Total population sampling.* Researchers are able to include everyone that is involved in the case under study.
- *Convenience sampling.* Researchers select those cases which are the easiest to access under given conditions. Often, due to limited resources of time and people, this is the only way to conduct a study, even though this is not ideal.

Examples of each of these types of sampling are evident in the literature. In their phenomenological study of young adult women exercisers' body self-compassion, Berry *et al.* (2010) used *purposeful* sampling to select participants based on their ability to provide in-depth, relevant information that would help them understand the research problem. This was informed by *criterion-based* sampling in that they sought out women who: (1) were between the ages of 23 and 29 years, (2) identified themselves as exercisers, (3) self-identified as having moved from being evaluative of their bodies to being more understanding and less judgemental towards their bodies, and (4) were willing to describe two instances where they experienced a kind, understanding and non-judgemental attitude towards their bodies and the criteria they used in this process. Jones and Lavallee (2009) also used purposeful sampling in their study of perceived life skills development and participation in sport to recruit a participant with strong life skills, who was willing to share experiences of life skills development. In making this choice they utilised *critical case* sampling in that the 'participant was not selected as a representative of young sports participants and young personhood in general. Rather, she represents a particular case of an athlete's response to organised sport to gain a more detailed picture of this phenomenon' (p. 38).

Purposeful sampling was used by Holt *et al.* (2009) in their interpretive analysis of life skills associated with sport participation. They also incorporated *criterion-based* sampling. The principal sampling criterion was that the participants were young adults who had played competitive youth sport (rather than recreational, national or international sport) during their adolescence. Holt and his colleagues also drew on *maximum variation* sampling in that they recruited participants across different sports in order to sample a range of experiences. Likewise, Monaghan (2001) used maximum variation sampling but also included *snowball* sampling in his study of bodybuilders, drugs and risk in which a participant recommended or introduced Monaghan to others relevant to his study.

In her ethnographic study of the use and meaning of alcohol among fans of Australian Rules football, Palmer and Thompson (2010) used a process of 'snowballing' with several key gatekeepers who gave them access into the social world of football fans. Likewise, in her ethnographic study of snowboarding culture, Thorpe (2012) utilised snowball sampling in which many of her interviewees were met during phases of participant observation, often via happenstance conversations in various locations in the field.

> For example, a conversation with an Australian female snowboard instructor on a chairlift at a resort in Canada led to an interview in a local cafe later in the day. During the interview, two of the interviewee's friends entered the cafe and, after introducing me and explaining that I was doing research on snowboarding culture and interested in talking to female snowboarders about their experiences, I had confirmed another two interviews for the following day. As this example suggests, the snowball method of sampling proved effective with many participants helping me to gain access to other key informants offering names, contact details (e.g., email addresses and phone numbers) and even vouching for my authenticity as 'a researcher who actually snowboards'.
>
> (Thorpe, 2012: 59)

In contrast, Holt and Sparkes (2001) used *total population* sampling as they were able to gain access to all the members of the football team that formed the case in their study of team cohesion. Stevens and Andersen (2007) used what might be classed as *deviant* sampling or maximum variation sampling in their study of erotic transference and countertransference in sport psychology delivery. Here, they focused on two

72

seasoned practitioners with long histories of working with athletes who represented extremes of the spectrum when encountering the erotic in service delivery and who provided them with highly contrasting experiences. One case study was about denial, suppression and repression of anything that hints of the erotic in practitioner–client relationships. The other case study was about a nearly unbridled reveling in the erotic with the client.

Kerr (2007) utilised convenience or *opportunistic* sampling to examine retrospectively the motivational and emotional experiences of an accomplished skydiver and how this experience changed as the result of a fellow skydiver's accidental death. More recently, Sparkes, Perez-Samaniego *et al.* (2012) used *convenience* sampling to explore how narrative forms combined with social comparisons to shape the cancer experience for an elite athlete who was a former student of one of the authors. Likewise, in her study of the sociological, phenomenological, existential and ontological impact of technology, in the form of running shoes, Gibson (2012a, 2012b) used both *convenience* and *criterion-based* sampling to select participants for semi-structured interviews. This was because he wanted to include runners from a variety of backgrounds and with different motivations, goals and experiences of running.

RESEARCHER ROLE

In qualitative research, the person and their communicative competencies are the main 'instrument' of data collection. Because of this, they cannot adopt a neutral role in the field and in their interactions with people during interviews or observations. They have to take on or are allocated certain roles and positions through a process of negotiation. This means that the roles adopted may change over the course of a study as will the kinds of information and ways of knowing that are made available to the researcher. The roles available to the qualitative researcher range along a continuum from complete observer (non-participatory, outsider and passive) to complete participant observer (participatory, insider and active).

> Between these extremes, the researcher is an outsider or an insider to a greater or lesser degree. The participant role being performed defines the researcher's social location with respect to the phenomenon of interest. You may be located more or less

on the outside of the phenomenon of interest or more or less on the inside. What the researcher is able to see, hear, touch, taste, smell, or feel is determined by participant role involvement.

(Jorgensen, 1989: 55)

Each role on this continuum has its advantages and disadvantages for data collection (see Chapter 4). The researcher as complete observer may sit on the sidelines undisturbed, and make detailed and extensive notes about a training session and the interaction between the coach and players. In this role, however, the researcher cannot interact with the coach or the players to ask them questions about their interactions and how they understand and feel about the situation. In contrast, the researcher as complete participant who joins in and becomes one of the players in the training session will get a different 'feel' for what is going on and gain insights into the interactions with the coach from the players' point of view. The researcher can also ask questions of the players during the action and access their thoughts and feelings in the comments they make to each other and their reactions to the coach. The disadvantage here is that researchers are too involved to take notes during the action and must rely on their memory of what they have observed, heard and experienced so that they can document this later after the action is over.

There are possible advantages when the researcher is already a member of the group or subculture that they wish to study. For example, access is relatively easy; the groundwork for rapport and trust is already established; the research is also useful for your professional or personal life; and the amount of time needed for various research steps will be reduced. As Glesne and Peshkin (1992) point out, however, being a member of the group you wish to study can bring its own problems. For example, previous experience with settings or people can set up expectations for certain types of interactions that might constrain effective data collection. That is, you may be confined by the role you already have and be unable to renegotiate this for the purposes of research. Given that you are already a member of the group and are used to how things operate you may also have problems in making the familiar strange for analytical purposes. Most importantly, you have to live with your colleagues and friends after the study has been completed and the results published! The pros and cons of researching in your own 'backyard', therefore, need to be weighed up as part of the pre-study decision-making process.

74

Research positions are not static and a variety of roles may be adopted during the course of a study. Researchers may begin by acting as a complete observer then begin to participate in some of the action in the field. As the study progresses, they may become more involved so that they end up operating as a complete participant observer for the purposes of data collection. As Jorgensen (1989) comments, 'Participant involvement may range from the performance of nominal or marginal roles to the performance of native, insider, or membership roles' (p. 21). For example, in Holt and Sparkes' (2001) study of team cohesion in soccer, Nick Holt started the study as a new graduate student playing for the university football club second XI, prior to getting promoted to the first XI. Due to his qualifications and experience he was then asked to help coach the team three times a week in the role of coaching assistant. At this stage he announced his desire to focus on the team for his research study and gained their permission to do so. Therefore, in this one project he inhabited the multiple roles of first and second team player, assistant coach and researcher. Atkinson (2012) noted similar shifts in roles in his ethnographic study of Ashtanga yoga as he developed friendships with the participants over time. According to him, he started to learn the most about Ashtanga when he stopped seeing other practitioners in the shala as subjects doing the practice, and when he had grown to know them as friends in a mutually constituted community involved in Ashtanga. With regard to such shifts in roles, Millington and Wilson (2012) note that researchers must be attentive to the dynamics that occur with being at once an insider and outsider, or when shifting between the two during a study.

Another key decision about the researchers' role in the field concerns whether they are *overt* (with the knowledge of insiders), or *covert* (without the knowledge of insiders). With the latter, researchers do not disclose the real reason for their presence in the setting and collect data without the permission of the participants. Often this role is adopted because the researcher thinks that their known presence might produce *reactivity*, due to the observer effect, which they can minimise through covert observation. Some researchers might adopt this role if they think that the group they want to study has something to hide or, they wish to examine exactly those types of behaviour and perspectives that are hidden from public view (Holloway, 1997). Although this type of research might generate useful results, for *some* it is deemed unacceptable on ethical grounds, particularly in SEH and educational settings (see Chapter 8). Beyond the ethical issues related to the covert role there are other serious disadvantages to the covert role.

In a covert situation, accessing knowledge happens in the maddeningly slow pace of everyday life. The covert ethnographer cannot expend too much energy or zeal to discover or uncover the machinations of cultural behaviour or the shared image of cultural reality. In other words, the ethnographer must live within the hidden identity to gain knowledge. To step out of character at any time would destroy the covert role so painstakingly put in place. Asking questions, posing hypothetical situations, or directing interviews and life histories are out of bounds to the covert fieldworker. Knowledge comes when and where the fieldworker can obtain it within the position of one who is part of the social network for ordinary reasons.

(Sands, 2002: 111)

In contrast, the overt and known researcher can ask questions, move in and out of role as required, and gain access to a wider range of settings and people as they can negotiate their roles in an open manner. In the study by Holt and Sparkes (2001), Holt announced to the team of which he was a member that he would like to focus on them to explore the fluctuating nature of individual and team peak performances over a season. Having explained the nature of the research, his role, the data collection techniques, and the ethics involved, all the members of the team gave Holt permission to proceed with his research. As a known researcher able to adopt multiple roles, Holt was involved in every team meeting over a season, both formal and informal. He was able to spend time with the team simultaneously observing their behaviours and interactions, special events and crises as well as collect data via formal one-to-one interviews and a reflexive diary. It is unlikely that this would have been the case if he had adopted a covert research role. Choosing to adopt an overt or covert role is therefore a complex decision-making process that includes weighing up both the benefits and risks that come with each role.

GAINING ACCESS

Often the *place* in which the research to be carried out is self evident in the question. If the questions relate to physical activity patterns in school or the ideologies that inform the delivery of health-related lessons in schools, then clearly schools will be the site of the research. Likewise if the questions revolve around bodybuilding and the construction of

76

certain forms of identity, then it is likely that gyms will be one of the sites in which the research takes place.

Given that certain activities only take place in certain spaces, this raises the issue of *entry* to the setting and *access* to the participants. According to Holloway (1997), gaining access means that researchers can observe the situation, read the necessary documents and talk to potential participants.

> Access to participants in qualitative research is a continuing process of ongoing inclusion and exclusion of informants and not a once-and-for-all procedure because the size of the sample is not always established from the beginning of a qualitative study but depends on the emerging concepts.
>
> (p. 20)

In terms of access, some sites are more open than others. As a member of the public you could go to the local park at the weekend to watch football games with a view to observing referee-player interactions on the pitch. In contrast, as a member of the public, you are not free to walk into a secondary school and observe students in their physical education lessons. To gain access to the latter there are a series of steps that must be followed. These include, at the very least, contacting the head teacher of the schools in question for permission to conduct research in their schools. Here, the head teacher is acting as a *gatekeeper.*

Gatekeepers, according to Holloway (1997), are individuals or groups who control information and can grant formal or informal entry and access to the setting and participants. They can impose conditions for access. They may be official, 'such as managers of an organisation, or unofficial, namely those persons who might have no formal gatekeeping function but power and influence to deny access' (p. 77). Gatekeepers can be found at all levels of an organisation and often the researcher will have to negotiate with a number over time. For example, the head teacher may allow access to the school but negotiations will still need to take place with Heads of Department and subject staff to gain their permission to observe their lessons as part of a process of *voluntary participation.*

Prior to granting entry and access, gatekeepers (quite rightly) will want to be informed about the purpose of the research, the possible outcomes and uses, and what their involvement in the study would mean to them in terms of time, effort and commitment. They will also want to know about any possible risks to themselves, the organisation and their clients, as well as any benefits that might accrue from their involvement in the research.

If the organisation and the people might benefit from the research then gatekeepers are more likely to grant access. Holloway (1997) notes the following reasons why gatekeepers might deny access:

- The researcher is seen as unsuitable by gatekeepers.
- It is feared that an observer might disturb the setting.
- There is suspicion and fear of criticism.
- Sensitive issues are to be investigated.
- Potential participants in the research may be embarrassed, fearful or too vulnerable.
- Gatekeepers may not know about qualitative research and see it as 'unscientific'.
- Economic issues – the research may take up too much time and effort for those involved.

Many of these issues can be sidestepped if the researcher is already a member of the group to be studied. As indicated earlier, however, being cast in this insider role has its own disadvantages that need to be considered.

THE TIME FRAME

Ethnographies require time, patience, energy and the willingness to immerse physically, socially, cognitively and emotionally in other's cultures . . . Neophyte researchers must reflexively analyse their own enthusiasm for social interaction with strangers, their ability to manage interpersonal stage fright, their desire to spend copious amounts of time away from friends and family members and their capability for sacrificing almost all of their free time.

(Atkinson, 2012: 33)

Qualitative research is necessarily time demanding and this aspect of the inquiry process needs to be given serious attention. This said, it remains difficult to know with certainty at the start of a project how long it will take. The tendency is to *underestimate* the time required. This happens because researchers produce 'ideal' plans for themselves in terms of their research design, but these are less than ideal in terms of the busy lives of people out there in schools, health settings and sports clubs. For example,

78

gaining access to a health setting may take more time than anticipated due to delays in your request reaching key gatekeepers and committees. Interviews that you have invested time and effort into arranging may have to be cancelled and rearranged due to unforeseen events in the participant's life. Having conducted an interview, time has to be taken to transcribe it verbatim (that is, word for word). Often, one hour of talk can take up to five hours of transcription time unless this is done by professionals (which is very expensive and beyond the scope of most projects unless they are externally funded). Once the interviews have been transcribed the analysis may take much longer than you anticipated as might the 'writing up' phase of the dissertation.

These time pressures should not deter people from conducting qualitative research. Rather, they need to be acknowledged and used to focus attention on what can *reasonably be done* within a specific time frame. Thus, while it may be reasonable for Monaghan (2001) in his funded PhD study to undertake field work in four hardcore gyms using time-sampling over a sixteen month period, this would not be reasonable for an undergraduate study. With the latter, it would be more sensible to focus on one hardcore gym using time-sampling for a period of three months. Likewise, for his PhD study, besides his field observations, over the period of a year, Monaghan conducted sixty-seven in-depth phenomenological interviews with a range of bodybuilders and weight trainers. Some of these interviews were held over several days, lasting in excess of six hours. For an undergraduate dissertation this would be an unrealistic expectation with a more realistic figure for in-depth interviews being perhaps five participants. Again, this figure is a guideline and not to be set in stone. The undergraduate researcher may initially decide that interviewing five participants will provide sufficient data only to find that one of the participants emerges as a critical case for the study in relation to the research question and so becomes the only participant to be interviewed not just once but multiple times and in greater depth. Whatever the outcome, the issue of time needs to be considered as a key pre-study task and not overlooked.

ETHICS

Whenever research has an effect upon the lives of people ethical issues will emerge. Given the nature of qualitative research ethical issues are pervasive and ongoing throughout the course of a study, from the kinds of questions asked, the kinds of techniques used to collect the data, the field roles adopted, and how the research is eventually written up and reported. Such issues and general perspectives on ethics are dealt with in greater detail in Chapter 8. In terms of a pre-study task, however, it is likely that at both undergraduate and postgraduate levels you will need to submit your proposal for consideration to a Research Ethics Committee (REC), an Institutional Review Board (IRB), or a Faculty Ethics Committee *before* you can start your study and proceed to collect data.

Such committees will be concerned with a number of key issues that include the following: informed consent and voluntary participation; anonymity; confidentiality; deception; right to withdraw; beneficence; and non-maleficence. Normally, your institution will provide a framework for you to deal with such issues in your submission, and will expect examples of key documents to be provided, such as, an informed consent sheet and a participant information sheet. In addition, professional associations of social scientists in numerous countries have provided ethical codes of conduct to assist researchers. For example, those working in the UK might find it useful to access the websites of the British Psychological Society, the British Sociological Association, and the British Educational Research Association for guidance on ethical issues.

Dealing with such ethical issues as a pre-study task operates at the institutional level and is a first-step in thinking about what might emerge in the field. Even this 'first-step' can present problems for qualitative researchers in their dealings with RECs, IRBs and other forms of ethics committee. For example, each of these expects researchers to develop ethical protocols that outline their study aims and activities and specify the risks and benefits to participants. As Damianakis and Woodford (2012) point out, however, when developing an ethically sound protocol, qualitative researchers might find it difficult to account for all aspects of an emerging design and predicting or controlling the research environment, which changes from participant to participant. They note, for example, that in qualitative research data collection typically involves face-to-face interaction with participants. Here, the researcher temporarily enters the participant's world and accesses experiences and reflections 'which might be highly sensitive and involve future or unforeseen risk for the participant and possibly others' (p. 709).

Franklin, Rowland, Fox and Nicolson (2012) raise similar issues with regard to the ongoing construction of informed consent that takes place

80

within the dynamic environment of the field. All this is way beyond the remit of the REC and IRB. As such, ethics in qualitative research is not a static practice and ethical dilemmas are not resolved in a once-and-for-all fashion just because ethical clearance is given by a REC or IRB for a study to commence. As researchers enter the field *process-related* ethical issues will have to be negotiated and re-negotiated along the way. The complexities of this process along with the various ethical positions that researchers might adopt in the field are the focus of attention in Chapter 8.

THE COVER STORY

According to Glesne and Peshkin (1992), pre-study tasks are not complete without a developed cover story. These are written or verbal presentations of yourself that you will be required to produce in your interactions with others. In essence, they deal with the questions that any sensible person would ask about your research if you are seeking their involvement. Varying levels of detail will be given in your cover story depending on the level of involvement and the needs of the person. However, all cover stories need to address the following as a minimum:

- Who are you?
- What you are doing?
- Why are you doing it?
- What will you do with your results?
- How were the study site or sites and participants selected?
- What are the possible benefits and risks to the participants?
- How will you maintain the confidentiality and the anonymity of participants and sites?
- How often would you like to observe or meet to conduct interviews?
- How long do you expect the observation sessions and interviews to last?
- How will you record your observations, interviews and other data sources in your study?
- Will you be judging and evaluating anything that the participants think, say or do?
- What will you do with your results?
- Why should I trust you?

SUMMARY

In this chapter we have focused on tasks that researchers can undertake *before* they actually enter the field and begin to collect and analyse data. While we signal these as pre-study tasks they should not be viewed as one-off events. They are starting points in the qualitative process and will necessarily be revisited once the researcher enters the field. For example, reacting to situations as they emerge and negotiating access to spaces and places is an ongoing process. Likewise, dealing with ethical issues as they arise throughout the study involves a constant process of reflection, dialogue- and decision-making. This said, we would emphasise once again, that giving time and serious attention to the pre-study tasks we have identified are likely to provide researchers with a secure foundation on which to base their studies and enhance their confidence prior to entering the field.

getting started with some pre-study tasks

CHAPTER 4

DATA COLLECTION

In this chapter we give an overview of various methods qualitative researchers can use in the process of collecting data. These range from the traditional (for example, interviewing) to more novel or emerging methods of data collection (for example, the visual and the internet). We begin with the most often utilised method of data collection in qualitative research, which is the interview.

INTERVIEWING

According to Holloway (1997), a qualitative interview is 'a "conversation with a purpose" in which the interviewer aims to obtain the perspectives, feelings and perceptions from the participant(s) in the research' (p. 94). Building on this, in their examination of the issue of 'truth' in interviews, Randall and Phoenix (2009) describe the interview as a relationship between two or more human beings. Furthermore, Kvale and Brinkmann (2009) suggest an interviewer is like a traveller on a journey to a distant country that leads to a story to be told upon returning home. Guided by their senses and historical knowledge, the interviewer as traveller wanders through the landscape and enters into conversations with the people she or he encounters, asking questions as they travel together, and inviting them to tell tales about their lives along the way. Accordingly, an interview can be usefully described as a craft and social activity where two or more persons actively engage in embodied talk, jointly constructing knowledge about themselves and the social world as they interact with each other over time, through a range of senses, and in a certain context.

There are various kinds of interviewing. Qualitative researchers tend to use one, or a combination of what are known as semi-structured interviews, unstructured interviews and group interviews. How each of these kinds of interviewing is utilised in practice will be influenced by the epistemological and ontological assumptions a researcher is committed to (see Chapter 1), the tradition that the qualitative researcher is working in, *and* the kinds of research question they are seeking to address (see Chapters 2 and 3).

The semi-structured interview

A structured interview is a highly standardised and purposefully inflexible way of interviewing. When interviewing, the researcher uses an interview *schedule* that means he or she asks all participants a set of identical pre-established questions in the same order. In contrast, in semi-structured interviewing the researcher uses a pre-planned interview *guide* to direct the interaction, and relies predominantly on open-ended questions. Although researchers do not ask the questions in the same way or form to each participant, the relatively tight structure allows them to collect the important information about the topic of interest while giving the participants the opportunity to report on their own thoughts and feelings. In this kind of interview the interviewer exerts some control, but in comparison to structured interviews, the amount of control they exert over what a participant can say and how they can say it is reduced. The strengths of the semi-structured interview are as follows:

- It gives greater control to the participants than the structured interview.
- It has the potential to allow the participant a certain degree of flexibility to express their opinions, ideas, feelings and attitudes.
- The participant can reveal much more about the meanings they attach to their experiences, thereby providing the interviewer with deeper knowledge about them than could be gleaned from a structured interview.

The weaknesses of the semi-structured interview are as follows:

- There can be barriers between the interviewer and participant that, at times, might mean certain experiences are not shared.
- It is difficult to conduct certain analyses, such as a structural analysis, as the structure is provided by the researcher, and not by the participant (see Chapter 5 on analysis).
- It risks losing some of the complexity of people's lives.
- It is more difficult to analyse than the structured interview.

84

The unstructured interview

According to Holloway (1997) the unstructured interview begins with a broad, open-ended question within the topic area, such as, 'Tell me about . . .' or 'What is your experience of . . .' or 'What is your view on . . .' In this type of interview the interviewer has a broad range of topics they would like to cover. However, ideas or issues raised by the participants as these unfold in their story are followed up as required. This involves giving the participant more control over the interaction than in either semi-structured or structured interviews. The strengths of the unstructured interview are as follows:

- It is good at eliciting and inviting participants' stories, their understandings of reality, their place in that reality, and the meanings they give to events, emotions, or behaviours in messy and detailed ways.
- It is useful for exploring a topic in broad terms.
- The lack of researcher control often allows for more spontaneous dialogue with the participant.
- It allows for unanticipated ideas, phenomena, affects, and so on to emerge.

There is, however, a price for a lack of structure and control, and the unstructured interview has the following weaknesses:

- The data is more difficult to analyse and to compare across cases.
- It is time consuming.
- It can produce a high volume of data that is not used for the agenda or focus of the researcher (that is, the '*dross rate*').
- It is difficult for an inexperienced researcher to conduct.

Focus groups

Guided by the researcher, a focus group involves a number of people collaboratively sharing ideas, feelings, thoughts and perceptions about a certain topic or specific issues linked to the area of interest. This kind of interviewing can be semi-structured or unstructured. It can be done face-to-face or online via the use of conference software. Online focus groups can be useful when participants seek anonymity or are from different time zones or geographical locations. For the most part, however, focus groups are conducted face-to-face, in a semi-structured style of interviewing. Often, but not always, participants are seated in a circle or semi-circle format in order to facilitate interaction and for all voices to be recorded. The researcher takes on the role of moderator (sometimes called a facilitator) whose task is to create a supportive atmosphere for the expression of personal, multiple, and sometimes conflicting viewpoints on the topic in question. The moderator introduces the group members to one another, introduces the focus of the group (for example, a question or stimulus like a documentary, story, or photograph), reassures them that there are no right or wrong answers, and facilitates the discussion not in an effort to get the group to reach a consensus, but to bring forth different viewpoints. Such facilitating, or 'steering', may involve periodically recalling the original focus of the group, prompting group members to respond to issues by others, and/or identifying agreements and disagreements among group members. It can also include reminding participants that there is no correct or single answer. Often, depending on the topic, and for ethical reasons, the group is reminded that what has been discussed should not be divulged outside the research setting.

Most studies consist of between four and fifteen groups. The size of each group typically consists of four to eight people. It is often recommended that there are no more than ten people in one group to ensure that all get a chance to share their views. Equally, if the group is too small group interactional dynamics suffer and there is a thinning of voices. In terms of group composition, it is common to aim for some homogeneity within each group in order to capitalise on people's shared (but often not the same) experiences. A focus group might, therefore, be comprised of participants with similar characteristics such as age, ethnicity, gender, or some characteristic important to the study. To explore some research questions, however, a more heterogeneous focus group may be required that includes a diverse range of participants. Other kinds of focus group that might be considered include a concerned focus group or a naïve focus group. The former refers to a group composed of participants who have a stake in the topic. The latter refers to a group where members do not have a particular commitment to the research topic.

Focus groups have been successfully used within SEH. For example, Harwood, Drew and Knight (2010) used focus groups made up of parents of young footballers in their study of the parental stressors in three professional youth football club academies. More recently, to examine the impact that stories of ageing told by older athletes might have upon young adults perceptions of self-ageing, Phoenix and Griffin (2012) carried out a series of mixed focus groups (that is, both men and women) with young adults to examine their perceptions of (self-)ageing prior to and following their viewing of a digital story portraying images and narratives of mature, natural bodybuilding.

Focus groups have the following strengths:

- They work well as exploratory studies in a new domain as the lively collective interaction can bring forth more spontaneous, expressive and emotional views than in most forms of individual interviewing.
- They allow for a dynamic dialogue among the participants and an examination of the social interactions between them. Indeed, with focus group data, researchers must remember to examine not just what a person or group says, but also the interactional dynamics (including the interactions of the moderator) that produce the talk.
- Focus-group participants have a high degree of control over the direction and content of the discussions. Power is diffused among the participants and the moderator during the interview.
- They can constitute spaces for validating experiences that, in turn, could be used to enact political practice or collective resistance. Focus groups can also create spaces in which participants challenge, extend, develop and undermine themselves and others in ways that allow for the proliferation of different perspectives, as well as allowing unarticulated norms and normative assumptions to be revealed. Thus the possibility for both individual and group empowerment and change is enhanced.

Focus groups also have a number of weaknesses:

- Some people might not wish to share sensitive issues and intimate experiences in a group situation and instead would prefer a one-to-one interview.
- Due to the interactive nature of the focus group one individual may dominate the discussion at the expense of others whose voices are not heard. In such circumstances, the moderator needs to be a skilful negotiator to diffuse this domination and draw out the views of quieter members of the group in a supportive manner.
- Bringing together a group of people on the same day and at the same time can be difficult and time-consuming. It can result in no-shows. Thus, it recommended to remind people a day or so before the date they are due to attend, and to over-recruit.
- Transcribing the interviews is very challenging due to voices

overlapping, cutting across each other, and so on. It can take from five to eight hours to transcribe one hour of talk.

■ Maintaining anonymity and the confidentiality of those involved can be problematic. This raises ethical issues (see Chapter 8).

Telephone interviews, computer-mediated interviewing and mobile interviews

Often each of the interviews described above are activated and engaged with in a face-to-face manner within an indoor space chosen by the participant or the researcher (for example, the participant's home or a university-dedicated interview room). There are, however, other ways to conduct interviews. These include, telephone interviews, computer-mediated interviewing and mobile interviews.

According to Hanna (2012), interviewing people over the *telephone* has numerous strengths. It is a cost-effective method of data collection that can provide physical safety for both researcher and participants. It can be a time-efficient way to ask additional questions or clarify points after a face-to-face interview. A telephone interview has the practical strength of allowing researchers to access and obtain data from hard-to-reach groups. It can be scheduled with some ease and all involved have the freedom to shift times at the last minute. This is particularly advantageous as research participants often lead busy lives and may feel obliged to meet if someone was travelling to meet them in person. Telephone interviews can also provide participants with an opportunity to disclose sensitive information that they might be reluctant to talk about in face-to-face interviews. However, a telephone interview can lose some of the subtleties associated with physical interaction. The absence of visual cues to questions can result not only in loss of contextual and nonverbal data. It can, moreover, compromise rapport, probing and the interpretation of responses. When interviewing using mobile (that is, cell) phones, signals can also be interrupted or lost altogether.

Computer-mediated interviewing, or what is sometimes referred to as online interviewing, is a form of data collection conducted through the medium of the internet. Rather than conducting research *of* the internet, as outlined later in this chapter, researchers use the internet as a *tool* to interview people: a tool through which to collect data. Computer mediated interviews can be divided into two main types: asynchronous and synchronous. *Asynchronous* online interviews are those that

88

do not require both researcher and participant to use the internet at the same time and are usually conducted via email. *Synchronous* (or 'near synchronous') online interviews involve both parties using the internet simultaneously to engage in a (*text-based*) 'real time' conversation using some form of 'chat' or instant messaging software. For example, synchronous interviews can be conducted on-line over FaceTime, Skype, in chat rooms, or by means of Skype messenger.

Computer-mediated interviewing, though rarely used in SEH research, has various advantages. Some forms, like e-mail and Skype messenger/video/audio interviewing, offer a degree of anonymity to participants that, in turn, might help them say things that they would not be willing to say to a researcher sitting in the same room as themselves. As with telephone interviews, interviewing through a computer also has an advantage over face-to-face interviews in that it enables researchers to interview people who have access to a computer anywhere in the world. In addition to extending access to participants, interviewing through technology may have generational appeal and thus help when a researcher wishes to examine a certain age group. Further, some forms of computer-mediated interviewing are self-transcribing in the sense that the written text itself is the medium through which researcher and participant express themselves.

There are, however, disadvantages to computer-mediated interviewing. Whilst time may be saved on travel, to have a good and in-depth interview can take double the time of a face-to-face interview. There is the risk that in cyberspace the interview loses focus. When working with a set of interviews simultaneously (e.g. on-line focus groups interviews), information overload can occur. Some people may also not be comfortable with technology. Another drawback of a computer-mediated interview is that, like with telephone interviewing, it can be deemed impersonal. Conducting an interview across cyberspace means that a number of non-verbal and verbal cues that might be relevant to the interview are missing. Some of these cues, such as intonation, can however be filled up with the use of emoticons. For example, a 'smile' could written as '☺' or ':)'. One should remember, however, that emoticons are not universal, nor can they capture the subtleties of many social cues. Further, it is important to consider that the effectiveness of interviewing, including generating rich and thick descriptions, depends on being relatively skilled at oral or written communication. Finally, computer-mediated interviews should never be seen as an easy option. Faster, cheaper and more technologically advanced interviewing is not necessarily synonymous with 'better' quality interviews. The research by Kerr and Emery (2011) on football fans in different countries provides an example specific to SEH that displays online interviewing in action.

The *mobile interview* is a means of interviewing participants as they move through space(s) (Buscher, Urry & Witchger, 2011). In mobile interviewing, rather than two or more people sitting down in one indoor space as is often the case when conducting an interview, the researcher interviews the participant as they move together through every day or selected spaces that either the participant or researcher chooses. The researcher moves alongside the participant and guides them or vice versa. Either way, the movement in and out of spaces gives multi-sensorial meaning by those involved as part of the process of shared travel that is context specific. For example, a mobile interview might be conducted as a participant travels to watch or play in a tennis championship, or as a coach goes about their daily business both with and without players in attendance. Here, the participants take the researcher to and through places and spaces that are significant to them. Moving through such places and spaces can provoke contextually meaningful stories that might not be produced in a 'sedentary' interview.

In these types of interviews the participants have more control over the stories they tell and the locations in which they are told. This can be useful when dealing with sensitive topics or areas that might pose a threat to a participant's sense of self or sporting identity. Mobile interviewing can also reveal the participant's mundane, everyday spaces that shape the interactions between participants and others in various settings. Finally, mobile interviewing is very much an embodied and multi-sensory activity. For example, walking around a sports complex together the participant might draw the researcher's attentions to the sounds and smells of various locations, the feel of certain kinds of equipment, or the tastes of certain kinds of refreshments made available. This multi-sensory data can be directly apprehended, thereby further expanding the researcher's understanding and insight of the participant.

Mobile interviewing is not without its problems. For example, this kind of interview raises ethical issues with regard to ensuring anonymity and confidentiality as well as the safety of both participants and researchers (see Chapter 8). Mobile interviewing can be difficult to conduct in noisy and fast-moving environments. Furthermore, the characteristics of the researcher might render some spaces and places out of bounds, such as the gender-specific changing rooms in sports centres.

CONDUCTING INTERVIEWS

Interviewing may appear to be a simple and straightforward task, but it is hard to do well. Given this, in the following section we will draw upon various sources (Atkinson, 2007; Gubrium & Holstein, 2002; Kvale & Brinkmann, 2009; Wolcott, 1995), as well as our own experiences of interviewing, to provide some general guidelines for conducting interviews.

The interview guide

In developing an interview guide, the following guidelines are worthy of consideration.

- Drawing on relevant literature and personal experience (if appropriate), generate a list of draft questions that relate to the research topic (see Chapter 3). Consider questions that address the topic in terms of experience, behaviour, context, values, senses and personal background.
- Reduce the list of questions. Discard those that don't really address the research topic or are similar to other questions on the list. To assist this process, think about planning the interview around a few big issues.
- Try to use open-ended rather than closed questions. Closed questions elicit 'thin' answers and invite a 'yes' or 'no' response. For example, 'Have you ever experienced a serious injury during your playing career?' In contrast open-ended questions are designed to encourage richer descriptions. For example, 'Please tell me about your experiences of serious injury during your sporting career'.
- Refine your questions. Work at phrasing so that the questions are intelligible, clearly worded, to the point, and understandable to the participant. Avoid using jargon, abstractions, or academic terminology. Questions shouldn't confuse participants but should rather be an invitation for them to talk freely and happily about something they have experienced.
- Group questions around similar themes.
- Structure questions by funnelling them in a way that keeps the interview going and opens up issues as the interview unfolds. It can be useful to begin with 'grand-tour' or 'ice-breaker' questions. For example, 'Can you tell me about your life as an athlete?' Such grand tour questions can then be followed with the set of 'mini-tour' questions.
- Place any sensitive questions in the middle or towards the end of the guide.

- The final set of questions, what might be termed a 'closing tour', invites the participant to fill in any gaps that might not have been covered in the guide. For example, 'Is there anything else you'd like to add about your experiences as an athlete that we haven't explored?'
- Ensure that you have not overloaded the final guide with too many questions. Often, asking less generates more and better quality data.
- Whenever possible practice using the interview guide by interviewing a friend or a colleague. After this 'pilot interview' or 'dry run', ask them to give you feedback on the kinds of questions you have asked. For example, which ones opened up the conversation and which ones closed it down? Which questions were hard to understand or were too vague? You should also listen to the recording of these pilot interviews to check on your own questioning style and where you might have jumped in and interrupted the speaker before they had finished what they wanted to say.

A number of scholars have chosen to publish their interview guide in the final research report. For example, Knight, Neely and Holt (2011) in their study of parental behaviour in team sport developed their interview guide around the following sections: ice breakers (for example, What is your name and how old are you?); transition questions that included talking about parents at games (for example, 'Have you ever seen examples of parental behaviour that you feel is inappropriate at sporting events?'), parents' behaviour during games (for example, 'How do you feel about your parents coming to watch you play?'), parents' behaviours during games (for example, 'Do you ever notice your parents' behaviour changing during games?'), parents' behaviour before games (for example, 'Do your parents do anything before games to help you prepare?'), and parents' behaviour after games (for example, 'What things do your parents do that you like after games?'); ending questions (for example, 'If you had a chance to tell your parents how they could help you when you are competing, what would you say?'); final activity (for example, 'To summarise this interview and check we understood everything, we would like you to help us create a list of 'do's and don'ts' for parents in youth sport').

In contrast to the detailed interview guide provided by Knight *et al.* (2011), Clegg and Butryn (2012) used the following more open-ended interview guide to study parkour and freerunning. The overarching question for the interview session was: 'Can you describe the overall experience of practising parkour or freerunning, focusing on the sensations, thoughts, emotions and meanings that are significant to you, as well as

92

how the element of risk is "felt" within these experiences?' Follow-up probes were contingent upon the participants' responses, and generally included one or more of the following:

(a) How have these experiences affected you?
(b) What was that like?
(c) What thoughts stood out for you?
(d) What physical sensations stood out for you?
(e) What emotions were you aware of at the time?
(f) What is it like to practice in a public/social space?
(g) What is it like to practice in a public space with people watching you?
(h) Can you tell me more about . . .?
(i) What else do you remember about that experience?
(j) How did that feel?
(k) How did that affect you? . . . How did that affect you long term?
(l) Have you shared all that is significant with reference to the experience? (Clegg & Butryn, 2012: 21)

As indicated in the examples given above, probing questions (or curiosity-based or expansion questions, as we prefer to call them) are used throughout interviewing. A probe is a technique used by a researcher to gain additional information from a participant and go deeper into their accounts, responses and stories. There are several types of probe that can be used. These include the following:

Detail-oriented probes: These are designed to fill out the picture of whatever it is you are trying to understand. For example, 'Who was with you?', 'What was it like being there?' and 'When did this happen in your life?'

Elaboration probes: These are designed to encourage the participant to tell you more about a particular point related to the interview. For example, 'Tell me more about that?', 'Why is that?', 'Can you give me an example of what you are talking about?' or 'Could you expand on that?'

Clarification probes: These are used to seek clarification. For example, 'I'm not sure what you mean by "burnout" – can you help by explaining it a little more?', or 'I'm sorry, I don't quite get it. Could you tell me a little bit more about it to help me understand what you mean?'

In addition to the above suggestions for how a qualitative researcher might prepare for interviews in order to maximise the collection of rich and useful data, we offer the following guidelines for enhancing the process with regard to what might be done before the interview, during the interview, and after the interview.

Before the interview

■ Contact your participant at least one day before the interview by phone and/or e-mail as a courtesy reminder, or to reschedule, if necessary, in case the participant needs to change the date, time or location.

■ Practice using your digital voice recorder (you may choose to use more than one), or computer if using Skype.

■ Think about what you will wear and how you want to appear to the participant. What will they expect you to wear? What assumptions will they make about you? How will they respond to certain kind of dress or appearance?

■ Be well organised on the day. Check again your digital voice recorders are working and you've put fresh batteries in them.

■ If the interview is a second or third follow-up interview, read and analyse the transcripts beforehand to formulate new questions or new topics for exploration suggested by the data and your preliminary analysis.

During the interview

■ Enter the interview in a courteous and respectful manner. Greet your participant appropriately. For example, don't assume to use their Christian name – wait to be invited to do so.

■ Try to make the participant feel comfortable and relaxed.

■ Think about where you will be seated so that your digital recorders can capture all voices clearly.

■ Once the interview has begun check again that any recording equipment is actually working!

■ Before the formal interview, explain once again the purpose of the study, the interview procedure and ethical issues like anonymity, confidentiality, data storage, and how the information will be recorded (see Chapters 3 and 8).

■ Where appropriate make notes in the interview to record, for example, non-verbal communication or the biographical objects in the room referred to by the participant (for example, family photographs at sporting events).

- Be an 'active' listener, which is a process of being attentive and responsive. For example, show the participant that you are listening through your bodily demeanour and your general attitude.
- When appropriate, seek to establish rapport and empathy in order to build trusting relationships so that participants are more willing to be 'open' about their lives. Be mindful of over-rapport and, in turn, becoming too familiar and overlooking matters that need to be problematised. Also be wary of attempting to empathise with participants by imaginatively putting yourself in the place of them. This is elusive and a problem as there is the risk of projecting one's own fears, interests and values onto the other (see Smith, 2008; Sparkes & Smith, 2012a).
- Where appropriate, consider engaging in what Dowling and Flintoff (2011) describe as *antagonistic* interviewing. This involves challenging certain stories so that space is created for alternative or more complex storylines to emerge.
- Don't ask too many questions at once. This can overwhelm the participant. Avoid asking either/or questions. This can set up the participant with limited choices and may inhibit answers.
- Appreciate the value of silence. Silence can be beneficial to elicit additional information and is crucial to the creation of meaning during the interview. The participant can use silence in an interview for a period of reflection, allowing them to provide richer and more detailed explanations.
- Keep reminding yourself of the research questions that inform the interview and the general purposes of the research project. This said, important information can come from spontaneous parts of the interview, where the participant has seemingly wandered 'off track'. Be flexible in your approach.
- Be aware that in any interview all the senses are used in creating meaning and understanding. Try to be aware of the sensorium in action and make a note of these wherever possible (see Sparkes, 2009a; Sparkes & Smith, 2012a).
- Watch out for signs of tiredness from yourself and research participant. Suggest a break where appropriate.
- At the end thank the participant for being involved, allow them to ask you any questions about the interview and project in general, and if required arrange a follow up interview.

After the interview

- Make field notes as soon as possible after interviewing and try to recall as much details of the interview as possible. For example: What kind of relationship do you feel you developed with the participant? How did they react to your questions? Did they appear nervous or open and at ease answering your questions? Adopt a reflexive stance to the interview process and product.
- It is courteous to contact the participant to thank them formally for giving up their time to be interviewed.
- You may also consider contacting the participants in order for them to give you feedback on the experiences of the interview process and ways that you might improve it for them.
- As soon as possible after an interview, transcribe it. There are various ways to transcribe data. For example, you might choose a routine transcription that is often called an orthographic transcription (see Figure 4.1) or a Jefferson transcription (see Figure 4.2). Routine transcription is verbatim (that is, word-for-word), but does not include the fine details of talk such as intonation or overlaps. In contrast the Jefferson transcription is a notational system that seeks to capture the subtle interactional dynamics of talk, such as laughter, micro pauses between words (marked by (.)), emphasis (underlined sounds are louder, capitals louder still), noticeable pitch rises (marked by the sign ↑), and the pace of speech (inwards (<) arrows show faster speech, outward slower (>)) (see Figure 4.2). Remember that transcription is a form of analysis (see Chapter 5).

With regard to the process of transcription, software is now available to assist with this and provide an alternative to typing by hand. For example, voice recognition software, such as Dragon 11.5, is available. When used

---

'Routine' transcription

1. I: What happened after your injury?
2. J: After breaking my neck
3. next thing I know I'm in a
4. helicopter, and the rugby pitch
5. below and I knew y'know my life was over.

Figure 4.1   'Routine' transcription

1. I: Wh↑at happened after yo' (.) in:jury?
2. J: (0.3) Afta breakin .hh, hh my neck (.)
3. next thing I know (.) I'm in a
4. helicopter, and u:m, the rug↑by
5. pitch below (0.2) and I knew (.)
6. >y'know< (.)
7. I: mmhm (.)
8. J: MY life was ov↓er.

Figure 4.2   Jefferson transcription

with a quality headphone, and after calibrating for the researchers' voice, voice recognition software can enable researchers to transcribe data by listening to the recording and then speaking aloud what the participant and the interviewer have said. As Perrier and Kirkby (2013) comment about their use of voice recognition software, this software allows the researcher to automatically transcribe what is said into a word processing file, which can be quicker than typing by hand. It also has the benefit of freeing ones hands to write analytical memos. However, as Perrier and Kirkby note, calibrating the researchers' voice can be time-consuming initially and sometimes technical accuracy is not good.

ENCOURAGING PARTICIPANT TALK

Interviewing should never be underestimated. Encouraging meaningful, rich and storied talk is not easy. It is a difficult craft or skill. During the interview there are a number of ways the participant can be encouraged and supported in sharing their views and ways of understanding their experiences. For example, drawing directly on the framework provided by Crossley (2000), Smith (2013a) asked participants (all of whom had suffered spinal cord injuries) during an interview to imagine their life as an unfinished book. He then asked them to divide their life into its major chapters, and briefly describe each chapter. Each person was asked to give a name to each chapter and describe the content of each. To further encourage talk, and invite rich life stories, Smith asked about who the characters were in each chapter, what the central theme(s) or message(s) of the book were about and what might future chapters contain. He also discussed with the participant what made for a transition from one chapter to the next and whom they would share the book with, hide it from, and say needs to read it. In addition, Smith asked how they could have told a different story about their life and what that other story could be.

Another way researchers can encourage talk is to draw on (un)solicited *personal diaries* and *drawings* (see Gravestock, 2010). They could also use *material artefacts*. These are objects that surround the participant (for example, running kit, letters, trophies placed on a desk, and postcards) or are inscribed on their body (for example, tattoos or piercings). Participant talk might further be encouraged through *graphic elicitation methods*. One of these is known as *relational mapping*. Here, participants are asked to draw a map of their relationships during an interview. For example, participants might use the structure of 'spider diagrams' or drawings with stick people to map their relationships within a sports club, coaching context or health setting. A further innovative form of graphic elicitation is *timelining*. This is a method in which a participant and/or researcher draws a temporal plot about a specific subject (for example, weight loss or happiness) in order to visually represent their experience of the subject matter as it unfolded over time. An example of this approach is available in the study by Sheridan, Chamberlain and Dupuis (2011) on weight loss.

Another technique to collect data and encourage talk is *photo-elicitation*. Here photographs are used to invoke memory and elicit accounts from participants in the course of an interview. It can involve the use of photographs produced and chosen by the researcher (that is, researcher-generated photo-elicitation). Alternately, it involves asking participants to choose their own photographs (that is, participant-generated photo-elicitation, or what is sometimes also called auto-driving or auto-driven photo-elicitation). A useful example of photo-elicitation is provided by Phoenix (2010a) in her exploration of the identities of mature bodybuilders. For her, this approach has the multiple benefits of helping people to remember key events and assist them in reliving their experiences during an interview as well as provide opportunities to ask participants about their experiences in different ways, such as asking about the process of deciding which photographs to take and the stories and events that are represented in the photographs.

Researchers can also consider collecting data and encouraging talk via *stimulated recall interviews*. This is an introspective research procedure that uses audio recordings, video footage, photographs, scrapbooks,

98

cards, or other aids to help participants to recall their experience of an event during post-event interviews. Either the researcher or the participant can produce these aids. They may alternatively work together or be assisted by others to help produce them. Following producing material, a unique interview guide is developed for each semi-structured interview to reflect the participants' personalised set of activities, challenges, emotions, and so on. In the subsequent interview, to stimulate recall about experiences and engage in deeper discussions about them, the recording is shown and questions asked.

An example in SEH of the stimulated recall method can be found in Cherrington and Watson's (2010) study of a basketball team in which members were asked to produce a personal *video diary* over a week about their day-to-day experiences of the club they were involved in. In their work on children's physical activity experiences, Harvey, Wilkinson, Pressé, Jooper and Grizenko (2012) used *photographic scrapbooks* developed by participants to stimulate recall and found that this method encouraged participants to speak vividly about their experiences. Further, in their study of white water activities, Mackenzie and Kerr (2012) asked participants to wear *head-mounted video cameras* and the recorded sounds and visual footage were then later replayed in a semi-structured interview to stimulate their recall. For Mackenzie and Kerr, stimulated recall interviews can be particularly well suited to investigations of highly mobile, fast, risky, spatially constrictive, or skilled practices that are otherwise difficult for researchers to gain access to in other ways. This method also has the potential advantage of enabling participants to engage with their embodied actions as they actually happened and facilitate reflection on the processes involved along with the context in which they are embedded in. Moreover, stimulated recall techniques like the use of head-mounted cameras have the potential to provide access to the range of senses involved in SEH and allow for the development of a more sensory form of scholarship (see Sparkes, 2009; Sparkes & Smith, 2012b).

One disadvantage of a stimulated recall method is that it can be logistically challenging. For example, participants need to be interviewed shortly after recording their experiences and this time constraint can create problems. Malfunctions with equipment can occur. Researchers also need to be aware that the memories stimulated are active reconstructions designed to meet the current needs of the teller in specific sets of circumstances (Sparkes & Smith, 2008a). As Randall and Phoenix (2009: 288) note, memory itself should not be considered an exact reflection of our life as lived. This is not a problem as, for them, at best, memories are constructions. As they put it, memories are 'facsimiles of actual events . . . By its very nature, and by necessity, our memory as a whole is a dynamic amalgam of fact and fictionalisation – a matter of faction, if you will'.

OBSERVATIONAL METHODS

Observational methods are often used within ethnographic research as ways to collect data (see Chapter 2). Observational methods are not, however, restricted to ethnography or exclusive to this tradition. Researchers operating in other traditions, such as phenomenology, narrative inquiry or openly ideological research may also harness the benefits of observational methods. Such benefits include enabling a researcher to examine peoples' lives in situ and life as it happens in 'real time'. Observational methods enable the researcher to record the mundane, taken-for-granted, and unremarkable (to participants) features of everyday life that interviewees might not feel were worth commenting on. This method can provide data on not just what people say they do (as in interviews), but also on what they actually do. Further, as O'Reilly (2012) argues, 'Participating enables the strange to become familiar, observing enables the familiar to appear strange' (p. 112).

Another reason for using observational methods is that these techniques can provide researchers with a contextual understanding of people's actions, interactions and emotions. Because observation assumes a long period of time in the field, this data collection method, more than most other qualitative methods, can enable process to be examined. Another benefit of observation is that the data collected can be a route to 'knowing people' rather than 'knowing about them'. Collecting this kind of data, especially when operating as complete participant as in Wacquant's (2004) study of boxing, can allow a researcher to 'get close enough to grasp it [for example, the culture of boxing] *with one's body*' (p. 7). Of course, none of this is easy. As Atkinson (2012) notes in his ethnography of Ashtanga yoga, observational work can be harrowing and involve feelings of awkwardness or shyness when in a new setting. Like all qualitative work, it requires energy, time and patience.

But just what is observation? Observation is the rigorous act of perceiving the workings of people, culture and society through one's senses and then documenting these in field notes or recording them through technological means. Participant observation, on the other hand, requires that a researcher not just observes, but also *participates* (physically, cognitively, socially, sensually and/or emotionally) in the daily lives and culture of those being studied. In practice, however, this distinction between observation and participant observation is more complicated. Here the classic typology offered by Gold (1958) is instructive. He suggests that a researcher might move through a continuum of observation and participation roles when using observational methods. As we noted in Chapter 3, these roles range in terms of how much the researcher actively participates in the field being observed. The roles are important as the one being performed defines the researcher's social location with respect to the phenomenon of interest (Atkinson, 2012). The researcher may be located more or less on the outside of the phenomenon of interest or more or less on the inside. Likewise, what the researcher is able to see, hear, touch, taste, feel, or smell is shaped by participant role involvement. Building on descriptions in Chapter 3, there are a range of roles to take when observing. These include:

- *Complete observer*: Sometimes termed the non-participant observer role. Here the researcher adopts a 'fly on the wall' approach and does not actively participate in the field but instead observes what happens and how things happen.
- *Observer as participant*: The researcher is only marginally involved in the situation. The advantage of this observation is the possibility opened up for the researcher to ask questions, to be accepted as a colleague, but not called upon as a member of the group under study. However, observers are prevented from playing a 'real' role in the setting, and this restraint on involvement can be a source of tension, particularly in a busy work situation (for example, a gymnasium or sports club).
- *Participant as observer*: Often the participant as observer has negotiated their way into the setting, and as observer is part of the sporting group under study. An advantage of this type of observation is the ease with which the researcher–participant relationships can be forged or extended. Observers can also move around in the location as they wish, and therefore observe more sites in greater detail and depth.
- *Complete participant*: At the end of the continuum, the 'complete' participant is part of the setting and takes an insider role. The researcher does not participate in the lives of the people in order to observe them, but rather observes while participating fully in their lives.

Although we have described these observer roles as discrete entities, they are not static. As depicted in Figure 4.3, the researcher may move between roles throughout the research project as and when conditions allow. In addition, as indicated in Chapter 1, observational research can be described in terms of the extent the researcher takes an *emic* and *etic* position. An etic position is one where the person does not participate in the culture. They remain, in a sense, on the 'outside', observing on the margins. In comparison, an emic position is one in which the person is an 'insider' within the culture. In relation to adopting an emic or an etic perspective researchers also need to consider whether they are going to operate *overtly* or *covertly* during the study (see Chapters 3 and 8).

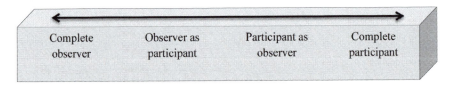

| Complete observer | Observer as participant | Participant as observer | Complete participant |

Figure 4.3 Continuum of role involvement

DOING OBSERVATION: PRACTICAL CONSIDERATIONS

To help guide observation, as Holloway (1997: 111) suggested, the following questions can be useful:

- The 'who' questions: Who can be found in the setting, and how many people are present? What are their characteristics and roles?
- The 'what' questions: What is happening in the setting, what are the actions and rules of behaviour? What are the variations in the behaviour observed?
- The 'where' questions: Where do interactions take place? Where are people located in the physical space?
- The 'when' questions: When do conversations and interactions take place? What is the timing of activities?
- The 'why' questions: Why do people in the setting act the way they do? Why are there variations in behaviour?

To contextualise these questions, and given that undertaking observation can at times be daunting and confusing, we offer the following points for consideration:

102

- Ask yourself 'who am I?', in relation to the setting.
- Think about the possible physical and mental risks to both yourself and participants (see Chapter 8).
- Reflect on the time, dates, and length of observation. For example, consider the time you have available to do a study (for example, four days a week, from 7.00 am to 8.00 pm, for three consecutive months), the daily length of time an institution or organisation stays open (for example, 7.00 am to 10.00 pm), the different people who might move through a particular setting (for example, shift workers, pensioners, unemployed, and professional sports people, or groups like mothers and toddlers, who all attend the same gym but at different times in the day), the dates of key events (for example, the Olympics or a local sporting derby), seasons (for example, the weather or the football season), holidays and religious occasions (for example, Easter), and how long might be needed to gain a deep understanding of a culture (for example, one weekend or seven months).
- Often, a researcher will only have a vague understanding of what is important at first. Accordingly, start out with a broad focus noting primarily descriptive aspects of the culture. Look for recurring patterns, including things *not* happening. As the research progresses, the focus narrows. Record observations in as much detail as possible. Holt and Sparkes (2001) provide an example of this movement from 'broad' to 'focused' in action. Their study initially focused on peak performance in football players. Yet, gradually, it became apparent that cohesion was heavily influencing individual and team peak performances. Therefore, their focus turned toward constructs influencing team cohesion: preparation strategies, player conflicts, and how players interpreted situations differently. Eventually, toward the end of the observation period, the focus narrowed further to examine player roles, game situations, relationships among players, and key incidents influencing team cohesion.
- Initially keep your eyes and ears open, and mouth shut.
- Observe the types of people (that is, actors) present in a setting. Over time, as you focus more, you may find a few people dominate a setting. These are important, but don't neglect the people in the 'shadows' or 'margins'.
- Observe action, reaction, and interaction. Action refers to not just what individuals do but also what they say they do. Reaction is how an individual responds to what is said and done by others. Interaction refers to the reverberating nature of action and reaction in process.

- Observe body language, including how people sit, non-verbal gestures, and their use of eye contact.
- Observe the place(s) and space(s) that people move in through time, including the layout and geography. Consider also sketching a bird's-eye view of the floor plans or outdoor environments to scale as much as possible, noting such features like furnishings, number of windows (if any), light quality, and wall colors. When useful, create diagrams of observations (for example, interactions in a setting).
- Observe when (in terms of time) things occur and in what order.
- Observe people's engagement and relationships not just with other humans, but also objects, technology, buildings, the natural environment, other animals, and so on.
- Observe material artefacts, goals and what people actually accomplish.
- Observe people's emotions.
- Observe and use all the senses – sight, touch, smell, taste, and sound.

RECORDING OBSERVATION

The traditional way to record thoughts and observations is through written field notes. Researchers might however also use a digital hand held video recorder, a head mounted mini digital recorder, a mobile phone, and/or a small laptop computer to collect and record observational data. The following are some points for consideration when recording observations:

- Begin broad when making field notes. In the early stages of being in the field record as much as possible. Later make your note-taking more specific as the research becomes more directed, focused, and selective. For example, as your investigation progresses, your research questions often become clearer, your writing becomes more refined and later centred on very specific issues.
- When possible record your notes whilst in the field, at the time of observation. Often, particularly when operating as a complete participant observer, in situ field notes are not possible. In this case, make notes in reflective 'down time' as soon as possible that day.
- Keep entries up-to-date by writing field notes daily; this is part of the essential craft of being a field researcher.
- Sketch the setting or take photographs of the setting. Draw diagrams and chart actions and interactions in the setting.

104

- Label each field note with a date, time and place.
- Sometimes it can be appropriate to develop an observational guide before going into the field. Fortune and Mair (2011) provide a useful example of this in their ethnographic study of the dynamics of a sports club setting.

VISUAL METHODS

The visual is increasingly been used as a way to not just represent data but also collect data. In a special issue of the journal *Qualitative Research in Sport, Exercise and Health* devoted to visual methodology, the guest editor Phoenix (2010b) presented a number of reasons why researchers might consider the visual. These include the following:

- Visual methods offer a different way of 'knowing' the world, which goes beyond knowledge constructed and communicated through written and spoken word alone. Visual material, like photographs, timelines, film, media images, drawing, and clothing, have the power to 'show' rather than just 'tell' things about our lives.
- Visual images can act as unique forms of data that have the ability to amass complex layers of meaning in a format, which is both accessible and easily retrievable to researchers, participants and audiences alike. The use of photography can increase participation and involvement of research participants and empower them in the research process.
- Thinking, writing, presenting and discussing with images can often make points more vivid and more lucid than written or spoken pose, and thus visual images are a powerful means to construct and convey key points, mundane aspects of everyday life, and emotions.
- Images can act on, in, and for us in powerful ways, shaping how are we able to see, how are we allowed to see, what is to be seen, what is not seen, and what we do and don't do. Given this potential power of the visual to *do* things, it would therefore seem sensible to examine them as a *topic* (for example, analyse the visual for what it might do) or harness the visual as a *resource* (for example, produce visual material to explore a particular issue). As part of this examination, visual forms allow researchers to ask different questions about SEH such as: How are we *able* to see? How are we *allowed* to see? How are we *made* to see? *What* is being seen, *how* is it socially shaped, what is its *affect* on and in people?

As suggested above, we can distinguish between the visual as a *topic* and *resource*. The visual as topic may include visual media images of the Paralympics or internet representations of female football players as the subject of analysis. The visual as resource to explore an issue, might include the use of visual material to collect data or produce representations of people. Drawing on Pink (2007) and Phoenix (2010a, b), we might further consider various forms of visual data that include the following. *Found visual data* is concerned with pre-existing representations that are already embedded within the field. An example of this kind of work, and how the visual is a topic for researchers, can be found in the work of Griffin (2010). As part of her ethnography of a UK-based women's only running group, she collected and examined a variety of visual material, including the front covers and images in women's running log books, promotional posters and pamphlets, newspaper article images of the women, and banners on the groups' website.

A second approach to collecting visual material can be classified as *co-constructed visual data.* Here, the researcher actively collaborates with others to create visual material together. Both the researcher and the other are *invested* in the research *process* as well as the *outcomes*. This kind of visual work fits the notion of participatory action research as a form of critical inquiry (see Chapter 2). Examples of co-constructed participant visual data can be found in the work of D'Alonzo and Sharma (2010) on the influence of *marianismo* beliefs on physical activity participation among immigrant Hispanic women, and research by Krane, Ross, Miller, Rowse, Ganoe, Andrzejczyk, and Lucas (2010) with female athletes on how they themselves preferred to be represented photographically.

A third approach to collecting visual data can be classified as *respondent-generated* and *researcher-generated methods*. For example, Cherrington and Watson (2010) used the medium of film to gather respondent-generated data in the form of diaries. In contrast, Kluge *et al.* (2010) as researchers created a video film to capture and represent how a previously inactive woman with little or no experience of playing sports became a masters athlete at 65 years of age. Another way to do researcher-created visual work or respondent-generated visual work is to use auto-photography.

Auto-photography refers to a method in which the person themselves takes photographs that represent their sense of self, emotions, or, for example, who they are in relation to a given phenomenon or topic (for example 'what health means to me'). Auto-photography can be a method used by autoethnographers (see Chapter 6) or be a personal project in and of itself. An

106

example of *researcher-created auto-photography* can be found in Atkinson's (2010) work on post-sport of fell running. He began to experiment with researcher-produced visual data as well as photo-elicitation following a conversation with a participant who relayed to him that the meaning of the practice of fell running is easily shown but not narrated. The participant, Atkinson noted, 'stimulated my sociological imagination further by asking, "Do you not know about running fells far more by seeing them and touching them as a runner yourself? Can you, yourself, put into words those feelings?"' (p. 118). Stimulated by this, Atkinson then chose to engage with visual methods as 'a means of digging analytically deeper into existential experiences fell enthusiasts regularly described to me, and which I experienced first-hand while running' (p. 118).

Participant-created auto-photography involves research participants themselves using the camera to document the images they choose. Sometimes the researcher will tell the participant to take pictures of whatever they feel is important in their lives. This can be useful, but it can produce images that do not offer anything meaningful in terms of 'answering' the research questions or the purpose that informs the study. Often, therefore, the researcher acts as a guide by asking each participant to take personally meaningful photographs about a specific question or purpose (for example what barriers do you face as a disabled person to being physically active). An example of how participant-created auto-photography can be built into the process of visual methodology can be found in the study by Phoenix (2010a) on mature natural bodybuilders and identity construction. Having conducted an initial life history interview with twelve mature bodybuilders, she gave each participant a disposable camera and invited them to take twelve pictures that say 'This is me', and twelve that say 'This is not me'. These photographs then formed the basis of a follow-up photo-elicitation interview as described earlier.

Griffin (2010, 2012) also used auto-photography in her ethnographic research (see Chapter 2) on the Women's Running Network. Again, to understand identity construction, she asked the participants to take a total of fifteen photographs, five depicting who they were (that is, 'me'), five who they were not (that is, 'not me'), and five that represented how they would like to be represented. To help further guide participants on this visual task, Griffin (2012) produced an auto-photography information sheet (see Figure 4.4).

Instructions for auto-photography task:

Describe yourself

To do this, I would like you to take 5 photographs that tell who you are. These photographs can be of anything, just as long as they tell something about who you are. These pictures should say, "This is Me!"

Describe who you are not

I would also like you to describe who you are not. To do this, I would like you to take another 5 photographs. These photographs can be of anything as long as they say, "This is Not Me!"

This is how I would like to be represented

Finally, I would like you to take 5 photographs depicting how you would like to be represented in 'society' (i.e., within running magazines, internet, promotional materials, ETC.). These can either be photographs of yourself, or of images that already exist in the public record that you feel represent you and your running experience(s).

To help you keep track, I have put a label on top of the camera/provided a checklist. When you take a picture of something that describes you, cross out a number under *Me* on the label. Similarly, when you take a picture that does not describe you, keep track by crossing out a number under *Not Me*. Finally, when you take a picture of how you would like to be represented (of yourself, or of existing representations), keep track by crossing out a number under *Represent*. Please remember, the 'Me' and 'Not Me' should not contain any images of yourself. In addition, whilst you are allowed to take pictures of other people, please take the following precautions for ethical reasons: none of the photographs should contain strangers, and permission must be granted by the individual(s) prior to the image being captured. In addition, none of these images will be reproduced in any reports (i.e., publications/conference presentations, etc.) emerging from this research.

Figure 4.4   Auto-photography information sheet (Griffin, 2012)

MEDIA

The *media*, such as newspapers, magazines, books, films and television programs, are popular sources of data in SEH research. For example, to help deepen her understanding of gender in snowboarding, Thorpe (2010) gathered and analysed data from magazines and films, whilst McGannon, Hoffmann, Metz and Schinke (2011) collected newspaper data to investigate the negative informal role in sport of 'team cancer'. There are several strengths of using media as data. Researchers can examine media texts as constructions in their own right and as representations about the corporations and institutions that produce them. Because many media resources have existed over a long period of time, these are a useful resource for looking historically at social change. Further, the media is easily accessible and a cheap way to collect data. Researchers can critically examine both what the media promotes and how it does this in various ways that connect to specific research interests in SEH, such as the social and political construction of the gendered and sexual body in sport.

Despite such strengths, much media research relies simply on the researcher's analysis of what is said or how things are communicated. This is classed as 'first wave' media research. For Millington and Wilson (2012), it is important to go beyond this when possible to also examine how audiences receive and interpret the same media analysed by the researcher. Do audiences receive and interpret the media in the same way as the researcher? Or do they receive and interpret it differently? Such questions, as part of the second wave of 'reception' media research, are of importance since people are not passive receivers of what the media says or shows, but are active interpreters who may resist, decode and question messages in the media as well as the researchers interpretation of them. Moreover, Millington and Wilson recommend that researchers examine how the media operates in the everyday lives of people, including the relationships between viewer interpretations of media and everyday social practices or experiences. This is the 'third wave' in media research.

Combined, the three waves have numerous benefits. For example, Millington and Wilson (2012) suggest that it moves research beyond simply *assuming* how media texts are interpreted. Interventions can also be fomented into the contexts in which they take place. However, the combination or 'triangulation' of the three waves does not mean that the researcher can pinpoint indisputable truths or provide knowledge of 'how media texts are understood with absolute certainty. Rather, it reveals *some* of the likely ways that media consumers interpret what they see and hear, and provides *partial* insights into audience members' lived experiences' (p. 144).

VIGNETTES

Vignettes are compact sketches of individuals or groups in specific scenarios. Some vignettes are written more as short stories whilst others are more like reports or descriptions. Vignettes can used to *represent* data (see Blodgett *et al.*, 2011; Sparkes, 2009). Also vignettes can be used to *collect* data by asking participants to respond to the vignette with what they themselves would do in a specific scenario or how they think either a third person or the protagonist in the story would respond. An example of vignette research (including the vignette itself) can be found in the work of Soundy, Smith, Cressy, and Webb (2010) on physiotherapy student's responses to a patient who has sustained a spinal cord injury through playing sport.

With regard to collecting data through vignettes the following are points for consideration:

- *Constructing*: Vignettes can be constructed from a range of sources including real-life case histories, hypothetical situations, previous empirical research, or in collaboration with participants during a study. The vignette can also take various constructed forms, such as a 'snapshot story' or a 'developmental story'. The former is a stand-alone, singular sketch of a scenario. In contrast, a developmental vignette is a story that unfolds through a series of stages. For example, in a developmental 'interactive' vignette participant's might select potential courses of action from a set of options given by the researcher. This could be done by hyperlinking a series of PowerPoint scenarios and making the choice of the succeeding slide dependent on the participant's reaction to its predecessor.
- *Presenting*: Vignettes can be presented on paper, DVD, audiotape, computer, in music or, for example, in photography. Where it can be presented to participants might include in an interview setting, in ethnographic fieldwork, before a sporting event, or in a lecture theatre.
- *Responses*: After presenting the vignette, participants are invited to respond to it. They may be invited to comment on how the vignette makes them feel, how they think the protagonist in the story might behave, or what they themselves might do in a certain situation by putting him or herself in the protagonist's shoes. A series of open-ended questions designed by the researcher might be placed at the end of the vignette to help guide responses in relation to the spe-

cific purposes of the research. Another option, as in a developmental vignette, is to ask participants to respond after each vignette stage unfolds rather than at the very end of the story.

There are various strengths to collecting data through a vignette. The vignette can be translated into multiple languages, thereby allowing researchers to collect cross-cultural data with relative ease in comparison to many other qualitative methods. Vignettes can enable participants to reflect on a situation or event that they may not have considered before, or which is highly routinised. In so doing, vignettes can generate rich data on topics that are rarely considered or taken for granted, yet remain important to understand. Further, by inviting participants to comment on characters in vignettes, rather than talk directly about their own experiences, sensitive topics can be examined in ways that appear less threatening and distressing to the participant.

INTERNET RESEARCH

Earlier in this chapter we highlighted how the internet as a *tool* can be used to collect qualitative data. It can however also be a site *of* and *for* scholarly study itself since, as Markham (2004) notes, the internet is a *place* where people spend time wandering, navigating, exploring, conversing, interacting with others they meet there, and exploring different forms of embodiment or body-self connections with others (for example, as Avatars in Second Life). The internet is a context to be studied in and of itself as well because it is a *way of being*. For example, the internet can become part of a person's self and shifting identities as he or she broadcasts daily activities via webcams or weblogs. It is lived through, used, reconstructed by people, and can affect their lives.

A number of approaches exist to conduct research of and through the internet. One approach is *virtual ethnography*, or what is sometimes termed cyberethnography, online ethnography, or netnography. Virtual ethnography is about conducting a study of virtual worlds. It is an online ethnography of internet sites wherein a researcher does not just observe the content of websites and how they communicate things, but often contributes to them as a recognised or registered member (Atkinson, 2012). Thus, a virtual ethnography involves researchers collecting data by actively immersing themselves in online sites, fields and communities, observing chat rooms, interviewing using web-based packages like Skype, reading blogs, Twitter feeds, and Facebook, interacting with photos and sounds, participating in e-mail exchanges, examining message boards, and so forth.

Another approach to researching the internet is *expanded ethnography*. This is a multi-site, multi-media, user-centered methodology that differs from virtual ethnography in that it focuses on *both* people's online worlds and their offline everyday worlds (Beneito-Montagut, 2011). Thus, expanded ethnographies have the added benefit of attending to people's everyday life and social interaction as taking place on and through the internet, thereby not only dissolving any 'real' versus 'virtual' dichotomy, but also highlighting how people use the internet as they go about their everyday day lives. For example, a researcher interested in football fans might examine not just football blogs or interactive message board threads of online football fanzines, known as e-zines (see Millward, 2008), but also how fans use their smart mobile phones on match days to communicate with each other.

Among the myriad of sources of data to choose from and work with when conducting internet research is 'blogs', or what is sometimes referred to weblogs. Rivalling web pages as the favoured medium of online self-representation, blogs are a form of internet communication in which an author regularly produces dated entries that appear in reverse chronological order (that is, earliest first) on a common web page. Blogs are characterised by instant text/graphic publishing, an archiving system organised by date and a feedback mechanism in which readers can often leave 'comments' on specific posts. Blogs are multimedia texts that can combine written text, photos (photoblog), art (art blog), video (vlogs or video blogging), music (MP3 blog), audio (podcasting), advertisements, and links to other websites. There are many different types of blogs that make up the 'blogosphere', including corporate, organisational blogs, and personal blogs in the form of an ongoing online commentary, diary, or journal (for example on sites such as Open Diary or LiveJournal).

To assist researchers seeking to use the blogosphere as a resource, Hookway (2008) raises the following issues for consideration:

- *Finding blogs*: Ensure they match the aims and objectives of the research and the questions asked. Scope initially for blogs by typing the phrase(s) related to the research topic (for example, exercise and cancer) into blog search engines, like Google Blog Search, Weblogs Compendium, Technorati, or Yahoo Weblog Hosting. Next, identify

112

the blog content management systems that host blogs. For example, a search of Yahoo Weblog Hosting might identify a pool of blog content management systems, such as WordPress, Blogster, Tumblr, Journalspace and/or Globenotes.

- *Sampling*: The search feature on blog content management systems like LiveJournal can also be appropriated by researchers to sample participants. For example, a researcher can find bloggers using this feature according to demographic information such as age and location as well as interests and hobbies. Keep a record of your searches as you go, noting such things as level of usage, gender, age and location of the author (if possible).
- *Assessment*: Evaluate the blogs to be included in the final sample by reading them in terms of appropriate criteria. Criterion for blogs to be included might include, the type of blog (for example hosting of personal diary style weblogs), the availability of a search engine that enabled identification of weblogs according to location (including country, county/state and city), demographic information of the blogger such as age and gender, and how many posts contained on a blog.
- Following finding, sampling and assessing blogs, *data collection* can progress by engaging in one or both of the following. Passive trawling involves reading through all blogs, including the blogger's entire back catalogue (which can be years), for how talk was performed, forms of discourse, what is said in terms of content, and/or different ages or concrete incidents. Active blog data collection encompasses soliciting blogs by selecting the relevant blog communities to advertise within. Once done, a researcher can email a copy of the invitation and seek permission to join the community and post. They can then seek interaction with bloggers by either leaving a comment on the post or by emailing and then, if successful, responding to the comment or email, thanking them for their interest in the project and inviting any questions.

Blogs as a data resource offer substantial benefits for qualitative research. A blog is often easy to access and provides a publicly available, low-cost and instantaneous technique for collecting substantial amounts of data. Moreover, the archived nature of blogs makes them amenable to examining social processes over time and doing longitudinal research. Like the majority of sources of internet data (for example, message boards), blogs also enable access to populations otherwise geographically or socially removed from the researcher. The global nature of blogs means they can be useful for conducting micro-comparative inquiry and cross cultural research as well as shedding light on processes associated with globalisation. Blogs may also on some occasions be used as naturalistic data (i.e. data collected without researcher involvement).

There are problems, limitations and dilemmas that, however, go with using the internet as a research context. For example, web pages can change or disappear from the web. This makes it difficult to contextualise data or understand how exchanges between people construct certain behaviours or emotions. When doing internet research it is also important to be conscious of 'the digital divide'. Access to the internet is not equal. Differences still persist across gender, age, economic status, education and ethnicity, and the extent of this difference varies by country. There are also ethical dilemmas associated with conducting internet research. Some of these are discussed more fully in Chapter 8.

SUMMARY

In this chapter we have focused on a number of different ways that qualitative researchers can collect data for their studies. Some commonly used data collection methods, such as interviewing, were highlighted. Less well noted and used methods in SEH, like the internet, vignettes, and timelining, were also attended to. This said, space limitations meant however that some methods of data collection, such as diaries (see Day & Thatcher, 2009) have been omitted. We would encourage researchers to consider the range of methods available to them to collect data, using one or a combination of these during the process of conducting their studies. But as ever, in qualitative research, no one data collection method fits all occasions and purposes. Choices about which data collection method or combination of methods to use need to be made in an informed and principled manner that should not just follow the trends of the time or stay within the boundaries of the well-worn and utilised.

CHAPTER 5

QUALITATIVE ANALYSIS

As Schwandt (2001: 6) rightly points out, 'If data could speak for themselves, analysis would not be necessary'. Data clearly doesn't speak for itself, and therefore analysis *is* necessary! Qualitative researchers analyse their data in a number of ways. In this chapter we introduce the main forms of analysis in use and also consider some emerging forms. Just as it is difficult to define precisely just what qualitative research is, so it is with defining what qualitative analysis actually entails. This is because many forms exist.

Given the diversity of analyses, researchers might be tempted to adopt *analytical triangulation*. This involves aggregating different analysis and triangulating the results from them. Analytical triangulation is however problematic. It rests on the myth that in aggregating analyses and triangulating the results the researcher can get closer to the truth, or counter biases or weaknesses brought by one method alone. Rather than analytical triangulation, therefore, researchers might choose to operate as an *analytical bricoleur*. This is someone who is well informed about a range of different analyses, skilled at using them, and adept at adapting analytic tools or inventing new kinds of analysis whilst maintaining an epistemologically and ontologically coherent position (Denzin & Lincoln, 1994).

To assist in the process of becoming an analytical bricoleur, and to provide a starting point for understanding analysis, analysis can be broadly conceived as follows: qualitative analysis is an artful and scientific interpretive process of meaning-making that begins at the outset of the investigation. It involves transcription, data management, immersion in collected data, a concern with what is in the data or how it is constructed, an examination of any possible interrelationships, and a reflexive awareness of the processes of writing and representation. With this broad definition in mind, in what follows we describe specific forms of analysis, how each might be done, and what the respective strengths and weaknesses are.

HIERARCHICAL CONTENT ANALYSIS

Content analysis is a generic name for a family of analytical methods that aim to systematise, reduce and interrogate the content of data by counting what is in it or by coding and identifying themes and category consistencies at a manifest or latent level (Hsieh & Shannon, 2005). At a *manifest* level, or what is sometimes termed a semantic level, the researcher examines what words or pictures appear directly in the text. They don't go beyond what has been said, written, or pictured and only focus on what is apparent. At a *latent* level, the researcher goes beyond what is said or depicted in a text to examine underlying meanings. For example, within the family of content analyses some require the researcher to count the frequency of words directly in a text, space measurements (for example, column centimetres in the case of newspapers), or time (for example, television time given to women's sport) and then draw references from this quantifying process about the data in question. Much media data (see Chapter 4) has been subjected to a content analysis of this kind. Other kinds of content analysis involve some form of coding.

As Saldaña (2011a) suggests, a *code* is a short, simple and precise key word(s) that represents and captures a segment of the datum's primary content and essence. The process of coding involves attaching labels to segments of data that depict what each segment is about. Each word or short phrase aims to symbolically assign a summative, essence-capturing, salient, and/or evocative attribute to a portion of data. The portion to be coded can range in magnitude from single words in an interview transcript to full pages of text. Saldaña notes that over thirty approaches to coding have been documented, including descriptive coding, values coding and dramaturgical coding. Which ones a researcher chooses for analysis depends on such factors as the tradition of qualitative research one is working in (for example, grounded theory), the types of data collected, the conceptual framework adopted, and so on.

A popular form of content analysis used within SEH is a *hierarchical content analysis*. The aim, when using this analysis, is to identify patterns in the data collected and explore the ways these patterns interplay hierarchically. A hierarchical content analysis enables researchers to compare and contrast *what* is in the data, divide the data into larger or smaller categories, and identify, coherently describe and order the material collected. As a result, general knowledge about a particular topic can be developed. For example, researchers who subject their data to a

116

hierarchical content analysis can reveal what a group of people has in common in relation to certain behaviours, affects, or experiences. On a more pragmatic level, this analysis also does not require the detailed theoretical or conceptual knowledge of many other approaches, such as grounded theory or narrative analysis. It is moreover a *codified method*. This is a type of method in which researchers are presented with a recipe-like technical account, or a procedural step-by-step formula, for how to do this analysis. As such, as a codified method, a hierarchical content analysis is largely accessible, particularly for those early in a qualitative research career. It equally allows researchers to present the data in a format that is cohesive and amenable for peer dissemination. An example of a hierarchical content analysis can be found in the work of Harwood *et al.* (2010) on parental stressors in professional youth football academies.

In terms of how to do it, a hierarchical content analysis proceeds through a set of steps. Five different terms are integral to these steps. Given that these terms are used in relation to other forms of analysis, such as Interpretive Phenomenological Analysis and grounded theory, it is important to offer a description of these before turning to how a hierarchical content analysis can be done. These terms are: theme, clustering, tagging, category and sub-category. Table 5.1 describes each term.

Table 5.1   Key terms in a hierarchical content analysis

Theme	A recurring pattern that conveys something significant about what the world means to a person.
Clustering	The process of comparing and contrasting quotes and connecting or separating quotes with similar meaning.
Tag	A label that is attached to a selection of data to identify it as meaningful piece of information. This is similar to *descriptive coding*.
Category	The collection, organisation and banding together of similar data and themes.
Sub-theme	Smaller units of similarly collected data.

The procedural steps involved in a hierarchical content analysis can be described as progressing in the following manner:

1. *Immersion*: this involves getting a sense of the database and becoming intimately familiar with it. For example, this can be done by reading the interview transcripts on numerous occasions or listening to the recorded interview several times from an empathetic view point. The combination of immersion and adopting an empathic position

is what Maykut and Morehouse (1994) described as the posture of *indwelling.*

2. *Search for, identify and label themes in each case*: search for and identify raw data themes characterising each participants' responses. To help with this, the raw data is first tagged to obtain a set of concepts representative of the information collected. Idiographic profiles of each individual can also be developed.

3. *Connecting and ordering themes*: independently cluster the raw data themes into meaningful categories that seem to connect and fit together. This analysis results in a cluster of raw data themes within categories of greater generality (sub-themes). These themes are then classified into larger, more inclusively meaningful clusters (higher-order themes and general dimensions), with each given a title that represents the themes contained within each category.

4. *Cross-checking*: the raw data themes and clusters are thoroughly examined again. The investigator or investigators who were present during data collection return to the original transcribed data and verify that all themes and categories were represented.

5. *Confirmation*: an investigator who was not present during data collection, but has experience in qualitative research, reviews the analysis.

6. *Produce a table*: the results are ordered in the form of a table or figure. The table or figure should be designed to display the hierarchical nature of the themes generated.

Along with its strengths noted earlier, which include developing general knowledge, a number of weaknesses have been identified with a hierarchical content analysis. These include the following:

- The researcher trades breadth for depth, resolution for scope, and thick description for thin description. In the analysis the messiness of people's lives, and the nuances and contradictions embedded within and across data, largely evaporate. Little is seen of the person in this form of analysis.
- It is easy to count the amount of themes or categories, and think that 'more is better'. Sometimes themes or categories that occur only a few times are highly meaningful and significant for understanding social life.
- Because the *whats* of data is the central concern in a hierarchical content analysis, when used alone very little can be known about the equally important *hows* of talk.

118

- When tagging, lifting small sections of talk from the data, or identifying higher order themes in it, data is often separated from the context of production. Data is disconnected from the participant's own contextual landscape in which their actions, behaviours and emotions are shaped. Thus, little is seen of the social contexts that shape what people say, do and feel.

GROUNDED THEORY ANALYSIS

As noted in Chapter 2, the tradition of grounded theory involves a specific mode of analysis in which researchers aim to generate or 'discover' a theory *from* data rather than impose theory *on* data. There are many good reasons why researchers might choose to use grounded theory. In their study that examined the delivery of video-based performance analysis by youth soccer coaches in England, Groom *et al.* (2011) used this approach as they felt it provided a meaningful guide to action. For them, grounded theory promotes analytical techniques, such as line-by-line coding and the *constant comparison method* (that is, constantly interpreting emerging data in relation to data already collected), that encourages researchers to remain close to their studied worlds and examine underlying patterns without taking off on theoretical flights of fantasy. The techniques of grounded theory are also helpful to develop an integrated set of concepts and categories from empirical materials that help a researcher to synthesise and interpret them, as well as show processual relationships (Atkinson, 2012). Another attraction of grounded theory, for some, is that as a *codified method* it offers a specified, laid down set of steps and instructions concerning how to do analysis, and what the final product should look like.

There are various kinds of grounded theory, including Glaserian (Glaser, 1978), Straussian (Strauss & Corbin, 1998), and constructivist (Charmaz, 2006) versions, and thus different ways to approach the analysis of data. Here we present a Straussian version of doing analysis. This involves the following steps as the researcher progresses though a number of different levels:

Level 1: Open coding
This initial level 'fractures' the data.

Conduct an intense line-by-line coding. This means labelling each line on each page of written data (for example, transcript). It can involve *in vivo* coding. This means coding by using the participant's own words. Keep codes short, specific, active and close to the data. This can also help to define *processes*, that is, the sequences of evolving action and interaction, in the data that otherwise might remain implicit.

Codes with similar meaning are linked together and, if these share common characteristics and key words, are organised into related features of a *concept*, which form the building blocks of any emerging theory. If the concepts cannot be grouped, as it represents a fundamentally different concept, a new concept is created. Whenever possible frame the categories in terms of *processes* rather than static entities.

Concepts are then examined in terms of their given *properties*. These are attributes, or characteristics that are common to all the concepts. Once each property of the concept is examined, engage in the process of *dimensionalisation* that involves arranging properties along a continuum.

Throughout open coding, engage in the *constant comparison* method. This is a process in which words, sentences, paragraph, codes, concepts, categories and literature are constantly compared with each other throughout the research. It is a way of continually checking that the emerging insights are grounded in all parts of the data and analysis.

Throughout also use *memos*. Different types may be used. These include operational and technical memos (about research design), discovery/ generation memos (concerned with the emergence of new ideas), speculative memos (concerned with conjecture), and theoretical memos (about the development of theoretical ideas). Memos serve multiple purposes, including transparency, clarification, category saturation, enabling reflexivity, and theoretical development. Charmaz (2008) recommends thinking about including as many of the following points in memos as is possible and useful:

- Defining each code, concept or category by its analytical properties.
- Spelling out and detailing processes subsumed by the codes, concepts, or categories.
- Making comparisons between data and between codes, concepts and categories.
- Bringing raw data into the memo.
- Providing sufficient empirical evidence to support definitions of the category and analytic claims about it.
- Offering conjectures to check through further empirical research.
- Identifying gaps in the analysis.

120

Throughout coding continually ask one of these analytic questions: *'What's going on here'* or *'What if'*. The former is a grounded theory question of the Glaserian kind. The claim is that this question permits data to tell the story. In contrast, asking 'What if' is the question a Straussian grounded theorist would ask. This means considering all possibilities, whether these are in the data or not. It involves asking specific questions such 'who?', 'what?', 'where?', 'how?' and 'when?' But no matter which approach is chosen it is important throughout the whole of the analytical process to remain open-minded to ideas.

Level 2: Axial coding

The idea here is to 'put back together' data fractured during open coding by relating categories to sub-categories, and specifying the properties and dimensions of a category. Axial coding can be undertaken in the following manner.

The data is first reassembled into *categories*. These are concepts that stand for a phenomenon. The set of categories is then examined as an entirety, to identify high-order categories and *sub-categories*. Relationships between categories and sub-categories are explored, connections between these are made, and concepts are redefined to form more precise explanations of the phenomenon. To help this coding for *process* it can be useful to ask, how does one code relate to another? Is one category related to another or does it exist separately?

Once relationships between categories are identified and verified tentatively, identify a *core category*. This is the central phenomenon or theme of interest around which all the other categories are related. To help identify the central phenomenon it is useful to keep asking what category appears frequently in the data and is related to many of the other categories that are emerging.

To help develop deeper understandings of relationships, and in turn theoretical development, consider examining the underlying *conditions* and *processes* associated with an emerging category. As in research by Hutchinson *et al.* (2013) on how people successfully change their physical activity habits, you might visually depict these conditions. Furthermore, to help in the development of theory, you might use and develop a *conditional matrix*. This involves visually depicting the relationship among concepts and identifying the conditions under which categories occur, and the consequences of their occurrence (a conditional matrix is used by some researchers at Level 3). Some basic questions to help identifying conditions include: under which conditions does the category or process develop and what follows these?

Consider using and developing a *paradigm model* (like the conditional matrix, this is used by some at Level 3). This analytical device focuses attention on the *context* and 'interactional' strategies that underpin the core category. Interactions are the responses that are taken to the core problem. Context is concerned with where a person is doing the category, when, and with whom. A paradigm model represents an attempt to encourage theoretical density within the emergent understanding. A good published example of this model can be found in a Strausserian grounded theory study by Bringer, Brackenridge and Johnson (2006) of coaches who had engaged in sexual relations with athletes or had allegations of abuse brought against them. Another example of a paradigm model in use can be found in Slater, Spray and Smith (2012).

Throughout, engage in the *constant comparison* method and keep memos. Also continue to remain open to new possibilities emerging from data and where necessary incorporate these into the analysis or emerging theory.

Level 3: Selective coding
This is the procedure that links all categories and sub-categories to the core category in order to craft and present a story of theoretical propositions. This level is sometimes also termed *theoretical integration*. Selective coding can be accomplished as follows.

Go over old memos or code newly gathered data, writing fresh memos as you go along. Abstract categories and concepts further during this level and develop them into the theory. Any theory should be traceable back to the data.

The constant comparison method is also used by comparing the core category, related categories and concepts with the literature in order to demonstrate the adequacy of 'fit', relationship and, where applicable, the extension of that literature through the research findings.

A final story needs to be told at a conceptual level, relating subsidiary categories to the core category, and capturing the theory. Some researchers display this in a final conditional matrix.

The end of a grounded theory study should reveal a substantive *theoretical model* of the studied phenomenon and not just a descriptive account of the data collected. At this stage, there should be evidence of *theoretical*

122

saturation. This type of saturation is different to data saturation, that is, the stage when no new information is gained through data collection. Theoretical saturation instead occurs only when no new ideas or insights important for the development of theory arise. The substantive theory produced must have explanatory power, show links between categories, demonstrate process over time, and be grounded in data collected. Many grounded theorists also suggest the theory should be displayed visually.

As noted earlier, a ground theory approach has a number of strengths. It also has a number of weaknesses that include the following:

- Grounded theory is very time consuming to do properly.
- Open coding is not something that can be easily learnt.
- The initial fracturing of data (that is, open coding) may lead, if the researcher is not careful, to the patterns in the data set being too fragmented and the 'whole' picture of the research lost.
- Equally, when dividing data into individual words, or coding each individual line, it is easy to 'drown' in the data and become lost within the details.
- Sometimes context is ignored and the theory is decontextualised from place, time and culture.
- The role of the researcher in the analysis is often overlooked and given insufficient attention. Their gaze is rarely turned critically on themselves. Set against this, Charmaz (2006) suggests ways that constructivist grounded theorists might address this lack of reflexivity.
- Many studies in SEH claim to do grounded theory, but on close inspection actually do not. For example, few studies in SEH implement the full set of complex procedures to produce a theory (Hutchinson *et al.* 2011; Weed, 2009b). Most often what is produced is a conceptual analysis and set of discrete themes instead of a substantive theory that is grounded. In other words, the analysis looks very much like a thematic analysis, not a grounded theory.
- Grounded theory does not lend itself well to other forms of qualitative research, such as phenomenological inquiry, as it has problems explaining lived experience.

THEMATIC ANALYSIS

A thematic analysis is a method that minimally organises and describes the data collected in rich detail by identifying, analysing, interpreting, and reporting patterns (that is, themes) within data (Braun & Clarke, 2006). In this sense, it is similar to other analytic methods that seek to describe patterns across an entire data set, such as a hierarchical content analysis and grounded theory. However, there are differences between a thematic analysis and other analytic methods that seek themes in the data. In contrast to content forms of analysis, a thematic analysis does not seek to quantify themes (for example, '77 raw data themes were found') or build thematic structures in a hierarchical tree-like manner. Moreover, whereas in a content analysis writing is not explicitly acknowledged as an analytic strategy, in a thematic analysis writing is openly part of the analysis (see Chapter 6).

A thematic analysis is a relatively straightforward and flexible form of qualitative analysis. A strength is that it highlights similarities and differences across the data set. It summarises key features of a large body of data. With a strong emphasis on interpretation, it has the potential also to push the researcher toward a deep, freewheeling, aesthetically satisfying interpretation of the data. A thematic analysis explicitly allows for social as well as psychological interpretations of data. Furthermore, a thematic analysis is not wedded to a specific theory. Researchers working in different traditions can use it. Another strength, according to Braun and Clarke (2006), is that the 'results are generally accessible to educated general public' (p. 95). It can likewise be 'useful for producing qualitative analyses suited to informing policy development' (p. 95).

Drawing on Braun and Clarke (2006), and as exemplified in SEH by Hall *et al.* (2012) in their study of Welsh rugby fans, the phases for doing a thematic analysis can be summarised as follows:

Phase 1: *Immersion.*

Phase 2: *Generating initial codes*: firstly, code across the entire data set in a systematic fashion. Next, identify and produce a long list of the different codes across the data set. Once all data have been initially coded, gather and collate data relevant to each code.

Phase 3: *Searching for and identifying themes*: here, refocus the analysis at the broader level of themes, rather than codes. This involves first sorting the different codes into possible themes. It then entails gathering and collating all the relevant coded data extracts within identified themes to produce a set of candidate themes. When doing all this ask how different codes may combine to form an overarching theme, that is, a common thread and 'meaningful essence' that runs through the data. You might use a 'thematic map' to help sort the different codes into themes. A 'thematic map' can be a visual representation, table, drawing, or mind-map of the themes thus far identified.

Phase 4: *Reviewing themes*: this phase entails two levels. Level 1 involves checking if the themes work in relation to the coded extracts. This is done by reading all the collated extracts for each theme, and considering whether these appear to form a coherent pattern. The aim during this level is to see if candidate themes appear to form a coherent pattern. But if the identified candidate themes do not fit, ask whether the theme itself is problematic, or whether some of the data extracts within it simply do not fit there. If the latter is the case, rework the theme, create a new theme, and find a home for those extracts that do not currently work in an already-existing theme, or discard these from the analysis. Once satisfied that the candidate themes adequately capture the contours of the coded data, and once a candidate 'thematic map' has been developed, move to Level 2.

At level 2, first ascertain whether the themes 'work' in relation to the entire data set. Secondly, code across the entire data set any additional data within themes that has been missed in earlier coding stages. After all this, return to the 'thematic map'. If the map works, then move on to Phase 5. That is, the data within themes should cohere together meaningfully, while clear distinctions between themes should be identifiable. If the map doesn't fit the data set, return to further reviewing and refining your coding until a satisfactory thematic map can be devised. By the end of this phase, the analyst should have fairly good idea of what the different themes are, how these fit together, and the overall story these tell about the data.

Phase 5: *Defining and naming themes*: this is a theme refining and defining phase that entails identifying the 'essence' of what each theme is about and determining what aspect of the data each theme captures. To help do this, identify and write the 'story' that each individual theme tells. Consider as well how the theme fits into the broader overall 'story' that is to be told about the data and in relation to the research question(s). It is also important during this process of refining themes to identify whether or not a theme contains any sub-themes (that is, themes within a theme). Sub-themes can be useful for giving structure to a particularly large and complex theme. Indeed, it is important not to produce a theme that does too much. A theme isn't supposed to be too diverse and complex. Once themes are refined, define each theme in no more than a couple of sentences and give a working name to each. Names need to be concise, punchy, and immediately give the reader a sense of what the theme is about.

Phase 6: Writing the report: this is another opportunity to refine the analysis as in the writing new ideas can emerge. In the report provide enough vivid data extracts to demonstrate the prevalence of the theme (evidence). Themes need to be embedded within an analytic tale that provides a clear *interpretation* of the data.

Like all forms of analysis, a thematic analysis is not without its weaknesses. These include the following:

- Like a hierarchical content analysis, when searching for themes the nuances and contradictions in the data can be 'ironed out'.
- It allows the analyst to develop themes but does not allow them to make claims about language use, or the fine-grained functionality of talk. It also tells us little about the artfulness of storytelling and the performative nature of language.
- There is a risk of the researcher getting carried away and producing an unfounded analysis. That is, one in which interpretations are not supported by the data, or, in the worst case, the data extracts presented suggest another analysis or even contradict the interpretations.

INTERPRETATIVE PHENOMENOLOGICAL ANALYSIS

Interpretative Phenomenological Analysis (IPA), as highlighted in Chapter 2, is informed by the assumptions contained within the phenomenological tradition. It has two complementary commitments: the phenomenological requirement to understand and 'give voice' to the concerns of participants; and the interpretative requirement to contextualise and 'make sense' of these claims and concerns. IPA is frequently used in a *codified manner* (Chamberlain, 2011). Very much like a hierarchical content analysis and a thematic analysis, it has a relatively straightforward set of prescribed guidelines for proceeding. This can provide researchers new to qualitative research with a sense of security, making the task of making sense of data less daunting. IPA is attractive to some as it is relatively sensitive to describing and exploring differences in experience across participants. The most frequent reasons offered for using IPA is that this approach focuses attention on and gives primacy to the participants' own understanding and experiences of a phenomenon experience. For example, to study eating disorders in sport, Papathomas and Lavallee (2010) selected IPA because it allowed them to explore athlete's subjective experiences of eating disorders in sport, and help to describe and understand individual's account of the meaning processes by which they make sense of their experiences of disordered eating. For them, 'the dual commitment of IPA to the principles of phenomenology and hermeneutics make it a good fit in terms of yielding rich participant descriptions and combining these with psychological interpretation. IPA offers a subjective, meaning-centered approach' (p. 358).

IPA is also valued given its idiographic commitment to examining a small corpus of cases. This said, whilst IPA values the study of a small group of people (like all qualitative research), there is variation when it comes to how many cases are needed for analysis. For instance, in order to say something meaningful and important about disordered eating in sport Papathomas and Lavallee (2010) analysed interview data collected from four athletes with eating disorders. In their IPA work on coaching and experiences of burnout, Lundkvist *et al.* (2012) interviewed eight Swedish elite football coaches who had reported high levels of burnout. Finally, in their IPA research on exercise adherence and dropout, Pridgeon and Grogan (2012) specifically recruited and analysed data from nine adherers (seven men and two women) and five non-adherers (two men and three women).

According to Smith *et al.* (2009), and Smith (2011), when conducting an IPA study there are several steps to follow:

1. Searching for themes in the first case
The analyst during Stages 1–4 works with the transcript of one individual. The first step involves reading and re-reading this person's transcript to achieve a sense of familiarity with the account as a whole (that is, immersion). During this individual case reading, comments are made in the left margin of the transcript to signal any early impressions of what is interesting or significant in the respondent's interview data. There are no rules about what is commented upon. The comments in the left margin are not attempts at 'open coding' as used in grounded theory, but instead 'loose annotations', 'unfocused notes', or what some call 'exploratory coding'. Comments can be descriptive (for example, the content of what the participant is talking about), linguistic (for example, how the participant uses language), or conceptual (for example, emerging questions in relation to theory).

2. Identifying and labelling themes

Return to the beginning of the transcript. Identify and label themes that characterise each section of the text. Record these in the right margin. Here, the initial notes are transformed into concise phrases that aim to capture the essential quality of what was found in the text. Academic terminology can be invoked here. The skill at this stage is to move the initial response to a slightly higher level of abstraction by finding patterns of expression which are high level enough to allow theoretical connections within and across cases, but which are still grounded in the particularity of the specific thing said. As in the constant comparison method of grounded theory, keep threading back to what the participant said.

3. Connecting themes

This stage is an attempt to introduce structure into the analysis. List all the emerging themes identified in stage two on a separate sheet of paper, and look for connections between these. Next, try to make sense of the connections between themes that are emerging. Some of the themes will cluster together. They will form clusters of concepts that share meanings or references. Here, like might go with like (known as abstraction). Other themes, however, will emerge as superordinate concepts (termed subsumption). This means that themes are characterised by hierarchical relationships with one another. Give clusters a label (name) that captures their essence. Clusters also need to be crosschecked with the initial transcribed material to ensure that these remain consistent with the actual words of the participants.

4. Produce a table

The table lists the themes that go with each superordinate theme, and an identifier is added to each instance to aid the organisation of the analysis and facilitate finding the original source subsequently. The identifier indicates where in the transcript instances of each theme can be found by giving key words from the particular extract plus the page number of the transcript. During this process, some themes will be discarded (the reduction of themes): those that neither fit well in the emerging structure nor are very rich in evidence within the transcript. Document emerging theme titles in the right margin: these need not be final but should enable you to articulate something about the concept identified.

128

5. Continuing the analysis with other cases

This stage involves looking for patterns across cases. One can either use the themes from the first case to help orient the subsequent analysis or put the table of themes for participant one aside and work on transcript two from scratch. Whichever approach is adopted, it is vital to note ways in which accounts from participants are similar but also different by identifying both repeating patterns and new issues emerging as one works through the transcripts. Once each transcript has been analysed, construct a final table of superordinate themes (salient themes representing shared higher-order qualities). Don't select themes simply on how prevalent each is within the data, however. Take into account other factors, such as the richness of the particular passages that highlight the themes.

6. Writing

This final stage is concerned with translating the themes into a coherent account. In this account the themes are explained, illustrated and nuanced.

Beyond those weaknesses of IPA highlighted in Chapter 2, the following are worthy of note:

- Concerns have been expressed as to how different IPA truly is from some other forms of qualitative analysis. For Chamberlain (2011) the emphasis on themes in IPA can lead to this research being indistinguishable from a content or thematic analysis.
- The focus in IPA on lived experience and the ideographic is not novel, and qualitative research in general claims to focus on these. As such, simply justifying that one has used IPA because it focuses on lived experience and the ideographic is problematic.
- The prescriptive guidelines offered by IPA coupled with the thematic emphasis in analysis can result in 'the phenomenology getting lost along the way' (Chamberlain, 2011, p. 50). Giorgi (2011) similarly argued that much IPA work does not have a phenomenological grounding and it can be difficult to see the 'phenomenology' in the analysis.
- IPA recognises that the bracketing of taken-for-granted assumptions about a phenomenon (epochē) is not fully possible. Yet, despite the emphasis on bracketing, there is a lack of discussion around the critical connection between the analytic method of IPA and the researcher's

engagement in analysis. The analysts' preconceptions, which shape any interpretation of qualitative data, are rarely discussed.

- Too many IPA studies describe themes, but lack sufficient or 'strong' interpretations of these themes (Brocki & Wearden, 2006; Chamberlain, 2011).
- Much like grounded theories, the prescriptive guidelines offered by IPA leads researchers to produce what the method suggests they should (Chamberlain, 2011).

Given these weaknesses, if researchers are to produce high quality interpretative phenomenological analytical work, then as Chamberlain (2011) recommends, they need to position IPA work much better, 'clarifying more carefully their underpinning assumptions and how they are using IPA as methodology rather than method' (p. 53).

NARRATIVE ANALYSIS

According to Frank (2012: 41), 'Narrative analysis raises the thorny question of whether there is a distinction between narratives and stories'. For him, there is a difference. He understands a narrative as a general structure – a template – that circulates in culture and which people rely on to construct the stories they tell and the intelligibility of stories they hear. Frank also suggests that what makes 'a narrative a narrative' is that in narratives one thing happens in consequence of another. It has a plot that sequentially connects events over time in order to provide an overarching explanation or consequence. Thus, people tell stories not narratives. Each story told is artfully driven by the person but is constructed from narratives which are supplied by the surrounding culture. For others however, there is no distinction between narrative and story. For example, Riessman (2008) views the terms 'narrative' and 'story' as synonymous. She suggests that narratives are stories that people tell. Each story 'connects events into a sequence that is consequential for later action and for the meanings that the speaker wants listeners to take away from the story' (p. 3).

Despite disagreeing on whether or not there is a distinction between 'narrative' and 'story' both Riessman (2008) and Frank (2012) agree that not all talk or text is a narrative, and what differentiates narrative analysis from other analyses is its focus on narratives. As indicated in Chapter 2, narrative analysis is an umbrella term for a family of methods that make sense of, interpret, and represent data that is storied in form (Riessman, 2008; Smith & Sparkes, 2009a, b, 2012; Sparkes, 2005; Sparkes & Smith, 2011). It takes stories and/or storytelling as its primary source of data and examines the content, structure, performance, or context of the story or storytelling as a whole. Accordingly, in contrast to grounded theory analyses, IPA, and thematic analysis, narrative researchers are wary of fragmenting the story and over-coding the data. They prefer to work with the whole story intact by analysing from the case so as to preserve the wealth of detail contained in sequences of talk.

In a narrative analysis the interest is not simply on what is said in a story in terms of content. The language and telling itself is also examined along with the environments that give shape to narrative content, structure and performance. That is, in contrast to IPA, grounded theory, hierarchical content analysis, and thematic analysis, in a narrative analysis the interest moves between *what* is being said and *how* and *why* a person or group tells and performs the story as they do in certain places (*where*) and under specific conditions at various times (*when*). For example, the narrative analyst is interested in how a story is put together to convey meaning, namely, to make particular points to an audience. For whom was this story constructed, and for what purpose? What particular capacities of a story does the storyteller seek to utilise? Why is the sequence of events structured that way, and not another? What narrative resources from the cultural menu does the storyteller draw on, take for granted, or ignore? Where do these resources derive from, and under what circumstances and conditions? Are there gaps and inconsistencies in storytelling that might suggest preferred, alternative, or counter-narratives? What does the story do on, for, and with people? How do listeners or readers respond to a story, with what affects, and on whom?

Narrative analyses have a great deal to offer. They are case centred, and can help researchers understand lives in very complex ways. Instead of reducing stories to inert material, left devoid of spirit, storied data is kept intact. This is particularly important given that we are storytelling creatures. Another benefit of a narrative analysis is that it reveals a great deal about the socio-cultural fabric of lives, subjectivity, feelings, agency, and the multi-layered nature of human experience over time and in different sets of circumstances. The analyst seeks to combine an emphasis on people as agents of their behaviour and a humanistic image of the person alongside unpacking the cultural discursive practices that people often take for granted, but which play a key role in shaping human experience and conduct. Further, given that a story is a prism through which meanings are constituted and communicated, an analysis of stories as a whole enables researchers to better understand the meaning-making processes used by individuals and groups. Another strength of narrative analyses is that, unlike many other kinds of analysis, they call on the researcher to commit to *unfinalisability* (Frank, 2012). This means respecting in analysis that stories always, like human lives that are spun through them, have the capacity to change and that as long as they are alive, bodies telling stories have not yet spoken their last word. Further, narrative analyses allow researchers to attend to both the *whats* of talk as well as the *hows*.

Thematic narrative analysis

One analysis that focuses on the *whats* of talk is a *thematic narrative analysis* (Riessman, 2008), or what is sometimes termed a categorical-content analysis (Lieblich, Tuval-Mashiach & Zilber 1998). This analysis allows the researcher to examine the core pattern in the life story by looking at the content of stories. An example of this is evident in the work of Smith and Sparkes (2004, 2005) and Sparkes and Smith (2003), who focused on what notions of time, what metaphors, and what types of hope informed the life stories of men who experienced spinal cord injury through playing rugby. In terms of how to do a thematic narrative analysis, a researcher can follow these moves:

Immersion.

Writing initial thoughts: write first impressions of the entire life story of one participant. Make descriptive exploratory comments about the data by, for example, underlining reoccurring phrases and highlighting on the transcript key events, characters, and turning point moments.

Identify key themes: this involves making connections across the participant's life story and attempting to identify patterns and meanings as constructed by him or her. To help with this process, code the data by looking for common threads in it. When looking for threads it can be useful to highlight specific words or phrases within passages, as well as entire passages of text. For example, a person may tell a story about a sporting injury that has a thread running through it around 'hope': 'hope' of returning to sport again, the 'hope' fuelled by past comebacks, and the 'hope' medical professionals offer in terms of successfully repairing the

132

body and making a return. To also help identify themes, when reading the data and thinking about the codes in more open ways the following kinds of questions can be useful to ask: 'What is going on here?', 'What does this theme mean?', 'What are the assumptions underpinning it?', 'What are the implications of this theme?', 'What conditions are likely to have given rise to it?', and 'What is the overall story the different themes reveal about the topic?' Note omissions and brief references may also be critical to the interpretation of a life story pattern. Provisionally name the emerging theme(s).

Tracking within a narrative: examine where a theme appears in the life story, any interactions and interplay between themes, and highlight the context(s) in which each theme appears.

Make conceptual comments: this involves moving away from the explicit claims made by the participant. Here, preliminary and tentative connections are made to various theoretical concepts that might be related to specific themes and issues raised by the person telling the story.

Name the theme and write the story: name the theme(s) and highlight the interrelationships between themes. Write a rich story that captures what each theme is about. Don't fragment the person's story in this process. Keep thinking about each theme in relation to the story told, including what the theme tells us about the *person* and the *cultural contexts* that shape them.

Compare and contrast: do all the above for each participant. Then compare and contrast the most meaningful themes. To help with this, consider using a diagram or other visual means to plot the similarities and differences.

Writing the report: represent the most meaningful themes across the participants and interrelationships among themes in rich and layered detail.

Structural analysis of narrative types

With regard to the *hows* of talk, one way to analyse data is via a *structural analysis of narrative types*, that is, of narrative *form*. In this analysis, the interest is on *how* stories are put together and the kind of narratives that are drawn on to scaffold and structure the story being told. In terms of conducting a structural analysis, the following moves are taken:

Immersion.

Identify the plot and create a storyline: this involves noting how events are connected, and how the story is told in relation to the person's past, present and future. It also includes asking such questions as, 'How is the story held together?' 'What narratives "out there" in culture shape how the story is being told?' 'What kinds of narratives are imposing themselves on the person?' Write down identified storylines, highlighting how each narrative is structured – put together – to achieve a narrator's strategic aims.

Naming narratives: cluster storylines into ideal narrative types and give these a name. For example, in their work on spinal cord injured rugby players and the nature of hope, Smith and Sparkes (2005) clustered the stories into three narrative types. These were the restitution, quest and chaos narratives as defined by Frank (1995).

Writing the report: represent the narrative types in rich and layered detail.

Performative analysis

Another way to examine the *hows* of talk is via what Riessman (2008) termed a *performative analysis*. As shown within SEH in the work of Smith and Sparkes (2002), Smith *et al.* (2009), and Busanich, McGannon and Schinke (2012), this type of narrative analysis is concerned with, and directs researchers' attention to, examining how talk among speakers is relationally and interactively produced and performed as a narrative. With regard to doing a performative analysis, the process involves a close reading of contexts, including the influence of the researcher and socio-cultural circumstances on the production and interpretation of narrative within a certain situation, such as an interview setting. The analyst 'asks "who" an utterance may be directed to, "when," and "why," that is, for what purposes?' (Reissman, 2008: 105). A performative analysis thus shifts from the 'told' – the events to which language refers – to include both the 'doing' and 'the telling'. Cultural context, audiences for the narrative, and shifts in the interpreter's positioning over time are brought into focus. Riessman further points out that language – the particular words and styles narrators select to recount experiences – is interrogated in fine detail, and not taken at face value.

134

Having offered a description of how several types of narrative analysis might be done, these descriptions should *not* been treated in a codified way. They are neither a discrete set of steps nor a formula to rigidly follow, like in IPA, grounded theory, or a hierarchical content analysis. In practice, narrative forms of analysis do not work like this. Certainly, narrative analysis needs to be rigorous. However, it is as much an art or craft as a science and is intended, as Frank (2012) argues, to encourage thought to move. For him, 'Too many methods seem to prevent thought from moving. Analytic or interpretive thought that is moving is more likely to allow and recognise movements in the thought being interpreted' (p. 73). Given this, the potential to encourage movement of thought should be considered another strength of narrative analyses.

Whilst a narrative analysis has certain strengths, it also has a number of weaknesses that include the following:

- Defining what is a 'narrative' in general, and especially in relation to the data collected, can be difficult. As a result, it can be hard to do an actual analysis of narratives.
- Whilst various aspects of the social nature of narratives are emphasised in a narrative analysis, the subtle interactional dynamics of talk is often ignored, including how stories get embedded and are managed, turn-by-turn, in everyday, social interaction. For instance, in a narrative analysis how stories can be invited ('Tell us about . . .'), pre-announced ('Guess what . . .'), or proposed ('Well, I have something to tell you about her') is often missed.
- Narrative analyses take a great deal of time; analysis cannot be rushed as the story told by the participant has to unfold at their pace. For those new to qualitative research, narrative analyses are also difficult because analyses purposefully lack a prescribed set of steps that should be rigidly followed.
- Narrative analyses risk reducing people's lives to simply a story. Stories inform life but life is more than a story. Researchers should remember that, for example, the body's corporeal presence is also important. They should as well recognise that stories do many things, but they don't do everything.
- A researcher cannot focus on both the *whats* and *hows* at the same time. Analytically, this is just too demanding, and ultimately unproductive. This said, the technique Gubrium and Holstein (2009) describe as *analytical bracketing* is useful. This is the process of

analytically moving back and forth between the *whats* and *hows* of narrativity. As analysis proceeds, the researcher alternatively orientates to the different aspects of stories. For example, they can first focus their attention on the *whats* of talk, analytically bracketing out any attention or concerns for *how* the stories were told and how they were structured. Next, the researcher can put their interest in the *whats* to one side and focus on the *hows*. The researcher then brings the results together to produce a complex picture of narrative life.

DISCOURSE ANALYSIS

Besides narrative analysis, another emergent form of analysis within SEH is discourse analysis (DA). Just like the terms 'story' and 'narrative', there are various ways to define 'discourse'. A story is one specific form of discourse in which one thing happens in consequence of another. But there are many other forms of discourse, including reports, chronicles, arguments, and question and answer exchanges (Smith & Sparkes, 2012). Thus, DA is different from a narrative analysis in that it has a broader focus on language; it focuses on more than a story. DA is also a fractured field, in that numerous approaches have been proposed and adopted within different disciplines. For example, there is discursive discourse analysis, Foucauldian discourse analysis, and critical discourse analysis.

Discursive analysis attends to the business that is done in talk. The analyst does not look outside of the text or talk. He or she only attends to features that people themselves clearly orient to in interaction with others. Further, rather than using data provoked by the researcher in an interview, for instance, discursive analysts prefer naturalistic data (Wiggins & Potter, 2008). This refers to research materials that would (ideally) have been generated irrespective of the researcher's activities. Examples of discursive approaches in action in SEH are evident in the work of McGannon and Spence (2010) on women, self and physical activity, Lafrance (2011) on leisure, and Cosh, LeCouteur, Crabb and Kettler (2012) on retirement and the transition back into elite sport.

Foucauldian DA understands discourse as constructing the objects and subjects of which it speaks. It is concerned with the discourses available to people within culture, and the ways in which discourse constructs subjectivity, selfhood and power relations. More broadly than discursive DA, it defines discourse as a group of statements or regulated practices that systematically constructs the objects of which they speak about and the ways they act. Discourse then refers to systems of representations and ways of knowing. In a Foucauldian DA the speaker is positioned in/by discourse. Attention is also drawn to the power of discourse to construct its subjects. Instead of power being a possession of certain dominant groups and as radiating downwards from one source, it is examined as relational and circulating. What matters is how a discourse is used within power relations rather than if it is 'bad' or oppressive per se. Analysts look beyond the text to put discourses into a macro context and connect them to wider social processes of power. Examples of a Foucauldian DA can be found in the work of Markula and Pringle (2006), and Thorpe (2008) on the various discursive constructions of femininity in the snowboarding media.

Critical discourse analysis (CDA) has many differing versions. Despite this plurality, all promote 'looking outside of the text or talk' to critically examine the social and political context of discourses. The different versions of CDA often share a concern with social power. This type of power is about the privileged access to socially valued resources, such as income, position, status, group membership and education. One important power resource to fuel and sustain social power is privileged or preferential access to discourse. Groups and institutions play a key role in controlling these discourses. Accordingly, power and discourse are wrapped up together and conceptualised as a possession of certain dominant groups or institutions. Instead of power being relational, in CDA it is something people or groups 'have' or 'exhibit' and which can be 'good' or 'bad'. Examples of CDA in SEH are apparent in Kelly's (2010) examination of newspaper reports of football and 'sectarianism' in Scotland and McGannon and Spence's (2012) study of how women's exercise and subjectivity is (re)presented within US news media discourses and the implications for women's health promotion.

Due to limitations of space, in what follows we will just focus on CDA. There are various strengths to CDA. Often the researcher makes their own political commitments explicit. By making these explicit, the reader is in a better position to judge their work. Further, according to Breeze (2011), CDA offers a promising approach for identifying and interpreting the way ideology functions in and through discourse. Its specific 'strength is that it bridges the gap between real language phenomena and the workings of power in society' (p. 520). It emphasises the way language contributes to, perpetuates and reveals the workings of power and ideology in society. Thus, CDA can be useful for those researchers who have an interest in how power works in society and what effects it has on and for certain people, groups and institutions in maintaining unequal power relationships. This approach can be particularly appealing to those working in the tradition of critical inquiry (see Chapter 2).

In terms of how to conduct a CDA, Fairclough's (2010) three-dimensional conceptualisation of discourse as *text*, *discursive practice* and *social practice* has been influential. This conceptualisation is based on the principle that texts can never be understood or analysed in isolation, but only in relation to webs of other texts and to the social context. The aim of this kind of CDA is to address social problems by identifying and interpreting the way ideology functions in and through discourse to contribute to and reproduce power. Ideologies are understood as systems of beliefs that the powerful groups use to maintain their position of dominance over other groups. Ideologies are conveyed and reproduced through language and the task of CDA is to expose ideologies and how these maintain hegemony – dominance – of a certain group and oppress others. Drawing on the type of CDA described by Fairclough the following are the steps undertaken in this form of analysis (also see Markula & Pringle, 2006).

- *Describe the content of the text*: examine the 'whats': 'what is in' the text. With regard to written texts, focus on the vocabulary, wording, grammar, syntax, sentence coherence, metaphors, similes, and so on. When analysing what is in a visual text, such as a photograph, focus on such matters like clothing, groupings, gestures, appearance, context of picture, colour, the camera angle, what the photographer zooms in on, and the type of shot (for example, close up or full body shot).
- *Engage in an intertextual analysis*: focus on the discursive practice by examining how people respond, use and consume the text. Examine also the context of the visual image and text (for example, when and where the image or text is situated in the newspaper, magazine, television programming, or internet web page) and the contrasts or contradictions between the visual content and text. Finally, examine what themes or discourses emerge.
- *Connect findings to ideology and power*: firstly, aim to reveal how texts are used for ideological purposes by connecting each theme

138

or discourse to a particular ideology (for example, healthism, disablism, nationalism) within which the text operates. Next, connect the ideological structure to power relations. To help with this, ask questions such as, what are the dominant groups that create a particular ideological structure through the text? What effects can they have for them and on others? Who are the powerful groups that benefit and stand to lose from such a discourse or representation?

Whilst CDA has many strengths it also has weaknesses. These include the following:

- It has been criticised for being an intellectual orthodoxy. For example, Breeze (2011) points out that there is the danger that CDA is treated as a reified product or a 'critical canon' that researchers adopt uncritically and un-reflexively.
- It is rare that critical discourse analysts turn their critical eye back on themselves and the work they do as people often in positions of power.
- Much CDA work has a predominantly negative focus. There is a strong emphasis on deconstructing a text and it is rare for social action to be reconstructed in a positive way.
- CDA rarely examines reader responses or the audience reception. Thus, we get to know a great deal about the researcher's interpretation of the text, but not much about how these texts operate in other social contexts.
- CDA also draws on a wide range of theories about language and society. These theories are not always clearly defined, and there is a tendency to draw on an eclectic mix of concepts from different intellectual traditions, not all of which are compatible. As such, it is recommended that researchers clarify the theoretical background to their work and readers of CDA turn a critical gaze on the theories used.

VISUAL ANALYSIS

There are various ways to analyse visual data. One possible way is via a *visual narrative analysis* (VNA) as described by Riessman (2008). Underpinned by narrative inquiry (see Chapter 2), this type of analysis focuses the researcher's attention on the production of the image, the image itself, and how different audiences interpret it. Despite being rarely used within SEH, VNA has a number of strengths, as illustrated by the work of Griffin (2010, 2012) on the Women's Running Network. Rather than just focusing on data as content as many other forms of visual analyses do, VNA is also concerned with the context of visual data (for example, the 'where' and 'when' of production), the 'how's of these (for example, how component parts are structured to create a visual narrative), and the reception of these (for example, how audiences interpret them). Attending to these in combination allows the researcher to understand the meaning of an image in more complex ways and develop a more richly textured knowledge of the data. A further strength of VNA is that it seeks to examine images as narratives. As noted in the earlier section in this chapter on narrative analysis, because personal stories are structured according to the cultural resources to which people have access, reading images as narratives facilitates insights into both the personal and cultural. It helps us to understand the functions that images can have, as actors, on people. As such, the analyst can develop critical knowledge of why images are produced and with what effects.

Drawing on Riessman (2008) and Griffin (2010), and expanding on their suggestions, the following is one approach to doing a narrative visual analysis:

- *The production of an image*: examine all selected images for how and when the image was made, the social identities of the image maker and intended recipient or recipients, and other relevant aspects of the image-making process. For example, in Griffin's (2010) study of aging and a women's only running group she used the following as data: website, brochures, pamphlets and posters. These were analysed separately from found data that was made by other people, such as newspaper coverage by journalists about the women's running group.
- *The image itself*: interrogate the images, asking about what the story may suggest, what it includes (and by association, excludes), how component parts are arranged, and the use of colour and technologies relevant to the genre (for example, a photograph, painting, or film). Examine also the interface of the visual and the textual. Draw any connections between images and some kind of discourse, including a written commentary, caption and/or letters of the image-maker that provide contexts for interpreting the image. This process can

140

help identify narrative patterns and strategies in the data. Identifying narrative patterns and strategies in the data as a whole can as well be done by locating where a pattern appears for the first and last time, the crossover between patterns, the context for each one, the characters, the predicament within each, and episodes that contradict patterns in terms of content, mood, imagery and evaluations (that is, tracking patterns). Concentrate on how the content of image is shaped by the context of its production. Carefully and methodically check and double-check for tensions and areas of disjuncture in order to refine emergent patterns and contextual matters.

- *Audiencing process*: as recommended in 'second wave media work' (see Chapter 4), examine how audiences themselves interpret the visual data. For example, inspect the responses of the initial viewers of the visual data, their subsequent responses, and any stories viewers may bring to an image or written text that guides viewing (for example, captions). Researchers might also conduct a focus group to elicit responses. If time permits, they could also move into the 'third wave of media work' and examine the ways images are used, or not, in everyday life via observation, the Internet and other qualitative ways of collecting data (see Chapter 4).

- *Interpret and write*: interpret images and texts for meanings related to research questions, theories, philosophical positions and personal biographies. If engaged in 'second' and 'third wave' media work, examine the similarities, differences and contradictions between audience interpretations and the researchers' interpretations. Keep asking critical questions about the images, including how and why was it produced this way. Throughout also write and re-write a story about the data. This can include writing about what the visual data shows, how the visual shows things, and what possible affects and impact visual material might have.

A VNA, although very useful, has the following weaknesses:

- It is labour intensive. Analysis can be daunting when one is saturated with seemingly countless items of visual data.
- When preparing for, and actually doing analysis, there is the matter of how visual data should be organised and re-organised. It is tempting to organise photographs images in a linear temporal sequence. However, this is not always ideal. This is because the ways people structure and experience reality may not be encapsulated in such

a temporal sequence (Pink, 2007). When analysing visual material, therefore, it is important to experiment with the order, playing with sequences and interpreting data along the way.

COMPUTER ASSISTED DATA ANALYSIS

In recent years, some researchers in SEH using traditional forms of analysis like grounded theory (for example, Bringer, Johnston & Brackenridge, 2006) and content analysis (for example, Camiré, Trudel & Forneris, 2009) have turned to Computer Assisted/Aided Qualitative Data Analysis Software (CAQDAS) to support their work. Among the programmes now available to assist researchers are Atlas.ti, HyperRESEARCH, MAXQDA, AnSWAR, TextSmart, Ethnograph and QSR NVivo. Several Internet addresses are listed below to explore CAQDAS packages and obtain demonstration/trial software and tutorials.

- Atlas.ti: www.atlasti.com/
- HyperRESEARCH: www.researchware.com/
- MAXQDA: www.maxqda.com/
- Ethnograph: www.qualisresearch.com/
- NVivo: www.qsrinternational.com/default.aspx#tab_you

These CAQDAS programmes vary in their complexity and sophistication, but the common purpose of each is to *assist* researchers in organising, managing and coding qualitative data. The basic functions that are supported by such programmes as NVivo include text editing, note and memo taking, coding, text retrieval, and node/category manipulation. Many now record a coding history to allow researchers to keep track of the evolution of their codes. The packages often incorporate a visual presentation module that allows researchers to see the relationships between categories more vividly.

CAQDAS has several strengths. According to Brown (2002), Davis and Meyer (2009), and Richards (2005), simplicity is one. For example, these programmes have very simple ways of coding, and allow researchers to streamline some of the mechanical aspects of cutting, pasting and retrieving data records. CAQDAS also allows the researcher to quickly and easily locate material and store it in one place. Another strength of CAQDAS is that by facilitating the recording of the source details for

142

coded data, including the date and time of the data collection, the steps in the development of the researcher's interpretation and analysis can be easily detailed.

In terms of how to use a CAQDAS program, as commercial packages, each one has its own book length manual, specialist language, on-line tutorial packages and professional workshops that describe the steps involved in running a program. Given this, we can only offer a brief outline of procedures involved in just one CAQDAS. This is NVivo. The following procedures for this system are drawn from Davis and Meyer (2009) in their work that, drawing on research on affective responses to sibling competition in sport, sought to compare 'manual' and 'computerised' data analysis techniques.

1. Transcripts are micro-analysed by breaking the data up into meaning units on a sentence-by-sentence basis through electronic simple coding. Meaning units are highlighted through dragging and clicking on statements relevant to the purpose of the study. The highlighted segment of text is assigned a code name through introduction of a free node (that is, simple code).

2. Codes are then used to turn data into emergent themes. As themes arise from collected data, NVivo allows for the categorisation of simple codes into more encompassing themes. With the assistance of the tree node option and minimal use of pencil and paper for personal notes, researchers can construct emergent themes emanating from the free node list. Here, simple codes are assembled into hierarchical categories by dragging, clicking and organising the simple code groups into complex categories (that is, umbrella themes) and their referenced sub-themes (that is, higher-order, lower-order themes). For example, in Davis and Meyer's (2009) work on effective responses to sibling competition the simple coding process of their study revealed five free nodes involving emotional support from a sibling competitor (that is, cheering, compassion, defending sibling, displaying pride, encouragement). These nodes were recognised as lower-order themes and were strategically placed under a more encompassing higher-order theme of 'emotional support'. By clicking, dragging and arranging these themes into hierarchical order, Davis and Meyer's data analysis resulted in a higher-order theme with a total of 45 references of 'emotional support'. Concurrent with the categorical capabilities of NVivo is the ability to visually represent these

emergent themes using the models option. Using the models option, the researcher can create a visual concept map (that is, hierarchical, circular, directed and orthogonal) that provides a breakdown of the emergent themes.

3. The constant comparative method, as stressed in grounded theory (see the section on this approach in this chapter), is next used. The categorisation process continues as more transcripts are coded, increasing the size of the higher order data categories by grouping the lower order themes that emerge. This process of grouping ensures that the themes in each category are distinct from one another.

4. Data is continually refined until no new categories or concepts can be extracted from the data (that is, data saturation).

Although the use of CAQDAS offers several advantages, a number of disadvantages exist:

- CAQDAS can be costly. Maintenance and upgrades can cost much also.
- There is the possibility of computer or electrical malfunction.
- Writing is also largely overlooked as a form of analysis in CAQDAS.
- Users of CAQDAS might be tempted to use all of the programme's functions rather than just the ones that would be beneficial in answering their research question from a particular methodological standpoint. Users can be enticed into believing that they must use the computer for every stage of the analysis. When this occurs, research becomes limited to seeing just the data and concepts that fit on a computer screen, and thinking shrinks to the size of the monitor.
- The accuracy involved in simple coding can result in an inaccurate representation of theme frequencies within the data as well as the double-coding of meaning units, blurring the distinctions from one theme and/or sub-theme to another (Davis & Meyer, 2009). Further, there is a lack of flexibility during coding. A lack of software-related flexibility during the simple coding process can mean that researchers need to spend more time adjusting simple codes when using CAQDAS than during the use of manual data analysis (Davis & Meyer, 2009).
- CAQDAS programmes can contextually distance the researcher from his or her data. For example, NVivo allows the researcher to use an auto-coding option through the use of key words. By typing in a key

144

word (for example, coping), the software will highlight and help with coding each use of the word throughout an electronic transcript. Yet this option is very problematic because it eliminates the social context of the word within the process of the interview or fieldwork (Davis & Meyer, 2009).

- It is easy when using CAQDAS programs to count the number of categories or themes, and think that 'more is better'. Sometimes a small number of themes or categories are highly meaningful and important for understanding social life.

In addition to strengths and weaknesses, there are also a number of myths associated with CAQDAS that are worth stressing:

- It is common to assume that the computer package actually *does* the analysis for the researcher. It does not. Researchers analyse, computers assist.
- There is the myth that CAQDAS is a qualitative methodology in and of itself (Davis & Meyer, 2009). Again, it is not. It is just a technique. Researchers cannot ignore their epistemological and ontological assumptions that underpin any analysis they engage in and the consequences of these for how data is understood, presented and judged (see Chapter 1).
- Another myth is that by CAQDAS inevitably enhances the validity of the analysis. It does not. CAQDAS holds no magical power. Not only is CAQDAS simply a technique used by a researcher to assist in the process of making sense of data, there are different criteria that can be used to judge the quality of qualitative research (see Chapter 7).

SUMMARY

In this chapter, we have given a flavour of the various ways that qualitative data might be analysed. In so doing, we explored both traditional and more emergent or novel forms of qualitative analysis and drew attention to why researchers might choose a certain kind of analysis over others. How each kind of analysis is accomplished has been considered and the strengths and weaknesses of each highlighted. We have intentionally not privileged one form of analysis over another. There is no 'best' analysis. As part of being an analytical bricoleur, analyses should be chosen and used in an informed, disciplined and principled manner.

As Coffey and Atkinson (1996) state, 'Qualitative data analysis requires methodological knowledge and intellectual competence. Analysis is not about adhering to any one correct approach or set of right techniques; it is imaginative, artful, flexible and reflexive. It should be a methodical, scholarly, and intellectually rigorous' (p. 10). We could not agree more and hope this chapter has not only confirmed such a view but has also acted as a resource to help readers with this process.

CHAPTER 6

REPRESENTING QUALITATIVE FINDINGS

Conducting qualitative research is not just a private affair conducted for the enjoyment of the researcher. The results or findings of the study need to be conveyed to others. For scientific or quantitative studies, there is a well-defined format for this reporting. The Sixth edition of the *American Psychological Association Publication Manual* (2009) provides over 400 pages of guidance on how to prepare and submit a manuscript for publication in their specific style. The conventional structure recommended is as follows: title page, abstract, introduction, methodology, results, discussion, multiple experiments, references, appendix and author note.

Given the philosophical assumptions and interests that drive qualitative forms of inquiry are very different from those that inform quantitative research (see Chapter 1), it is not surprising that they report their work differently, draw upon different discourses, and utilise different rhetorical strategies to persuade the reader that their accounts are authoritative.

STRUCTURING A QUALITATIVE REPORT

For Holloway (1997), even though qualitative writing may differ substantially from a quantitative report, she believes that commonalities exist and suggests that qualitative researchers organise their dissertation or thesis in the following sequence.

Title
Abstract
Acknowledgement and dedication
Table of contents
Introduction
    Background and justification of the study
    The aim of the research
    Initial *literature review* (or overview of the literature)

Methodology and *methods*
Description and justification of methodology
(Including type of theoretical framework such as *symbolic inter-actionism* or *phenomenology*)
The sample and the setting
Specific procedures for data collection
Data analysis
Ethics
Findings/results and discussion (The findings and discussion are the most important elements of the final write-up and in consequence contain more words)
Conclusion and implications (Implications and/or recommendations are necessary for applied research in the professions for instance)
References
Appendices

(Holloway, 1997: 140–141)

Pitney and Parker (2009) suggest that regardless of the type of qualitative report (thesis, dissertation, or journal article) the following components should be included in every report.

1. Introduction
2. Review of literature
3. Methods
4. Results
5. Discussion
6. Conclusions

These and other authors give excellent advice on what should be included in the various sections of a qualitative report. Accordingly, we will only touch on various sections in what follows:

Title: A good title seizes the readers' attention whilst informing them of the essence of your research project. On this issue, Silverman (2000) notes his preference for a two-part title: a snappy main title, often using the present participle to indicate activity; and a more descriptive subtitle. Given that others will search and access your work via electronic databases it is important that the key words describing the nature and content of your inquiry are suitably combined in the title.

148

Abstract: Silverman (2000, p. 222) suggests that this should cover the following.

- Your research problem.
- Why that problem is important and worth studying.
- Your data and methods.
- Your main findings.
- Their implications in the light of other research.

Smith *et al.* (2009: 111) note that the abstract of a paper using interpretive phenomenological analysis should concisely summarise the content for the benefit of someone who knows nothing about what you have done. The abstract should include the following.

- Define the research question/problem and state why it is important.
- Introduce the general subject matter.
- Describe your sample.
- Outline the data collection and analysis methods, and explain *why* you used them.
- Summarise what you found.
- Explain what you think this means, and how it relates to other research or practice.

A word limit is often set for an abstract in journals which needs to be adhered to. For dissertations and theses, the institution is likely to set a word limit for the abstract.

Introduction: This should answer the question: what is this thesis or paper about? Silverman (2000: 223–224) suggests this is answered by explaining the following.

- Why you have chosen this topic rather than any other, for example, either because it has been neglected or because it is much discussed but not properly or fully.
- Why this topic interests you.
- The kind of research approach or academic discipline you will utilise.
- Your research questions or problems.

Pitney and Parker (2009) note that in addressing such questions, the introduction should ease the reader into your topic and lead them logically toward your purpose statement and research questions (see Chapter

3). They state, 'it provides a context for your research that allows readers to understand what you intend to accomplish and why your study will be significant, or how it will contribute to the existing body of knowledge' (p. 87). Note: An introduction is *not* a literature review.

Literature review: This was discussed in detail in Chapter 3 under 'prestudy tasks.' Suffice to say that, following Silverman (2000: 227), the literature review should address the following questions.

- What do we already know about the topic?
- What do we have to say critically about what is already known?
- Has anyone else ever done anything exactly the same?
- Has anyone else done anything that is related?
- Where does your work fit in with what has gone before?
- Why is your research worth doing in the light of what has already been done?

Remember that the literature review needs to be focused on studies relevant to your research questions and problems. Avoid tedious and irrelevant description. Critique the most relevant studies rather than just report them in the form of a laundry list of references As Pitney and Parker (2009) recommend, work concepts together into a rich narrative as part of the literature review and organise the review around themes identified from a critical reading of key articles and texts. As indicated in Chapter 3, the literature review will almost certainly be modified as the study progresses and issues emerge during your engagement in the field and as the data are analysed. Realistically, the literature review may be the *last* section you complete in your thesis.

Methods: Silverman (2000: 235) suggests that the following answers need to be addressed in this part of your thesis or paper.

- How did you go about your research?
- What overall strategy did you adopt and why?
- What design and techniques did you use?
- Why these and not others?

Likewise, Pitney and Parker (2009) propose that the methods section should cover the following aspects of your study.

- Who were the participants and how were they selected?
- What procedures were used to identify and recruit participants?

150

- What were the participants required to do?
- Where was the data be collected, what was collected, and why?
- How was the data analysed?
- How was the trustworthiness of the data assured?

How these questions are answered can vary depending on the qualitative tradition being used. In the methods section of their paper that utilises an *ethnographic* approach to explore organisational functioning in a national sport organisation, Wagstaff *et al.* (2012) discuss method under the following sub-headings:

Ethnographic inquiry
Participants and organisation
Ethnographic techniques
    Observation
    Field notes and reflexive diary
    Interviews and informal communications
Analysis and ethnographic product

In contrast, in their *phenomenological* analysis on coping effectiveness in golf, Nicholls, Holt and Polman (2005) included the following in their methods section:

Methodology
Participants
Procedure
Data collection
    Interview protocol
    The interview schedule
Data analysis
Validity/Trustworthiness/Goodness Criteria
    Bracketing
    Member-checking

Different again, in their *grounded theory* study of elite male table tennis players' activity during matches, Poizat, Saury and Durand (2006) included the following in their methods section:

Participants and procedure
Data collection
Data processing
    Generating match logs
    Labelling the elementary units of meaning

> Identifying meaningful structures in the course of action
> Construction of a grounded theory of elite table tennis players' activity during matches
Trustworthiness of the data and analysis.

These examples illustrate that what is included in the methods section and how key issues are dealt with can vary depending on the topic, the research tradition, and even the journal chosen as an outlet for publication. There is no one way to construct a methods section for your study and variations will occur depending on context and purpose.

Results: For most readers this section of the article or thesis is the most interesting feature. It tells the reader what you found out in your study in relation to your research questions and the issues identified in the literature review. Pitney and Parker (2009: 98) make the following observation about reporting the results of a study, 'you have the opportunity to present your position, explain the evidence you have collected to answer your research questions, help others gain tremendous insights about your investigation, and, most importantly, highlight the voices of the participants'.

How the results are presented will vary according to the tradition the researcher is working in, where the work is being published, and for whom. It is crucial that relevant and sufficient evidence (of whatever kind) is presented in the results section to support any claims that are made, however. For example, in their ethnographic study, Wagstaff *et al.* (2012) state that, 'findings are told through the participants' own voices with rich in-depth quotations, supplemented by researcher reflections to give a pen-portrait of the factors that promote positive interpersonal and psychosocial operations in the sport organization' (p. 32). Detailed descriptions are provided of organisational settings and interactions as observed by the researcher along with his own experiences of operating within the settings. Extensive quotations from formal interviews and informal communications with participants are included to support the claims made about the relevance of key themes and the connections between them.

Interweaving direct quotes from participants along with observations made by the researcher in the results section is a traditional strategy for qualitative researchers. Each of these constitutes the 'raw data' of the study and brings the results section to life for the reader so that they can see how emergent themes are supported in the analysis. Just how

152

participant quotes are used, raises the issue of voices in the findings and how they are balanced. Pitney and Parker (2009) consider the following options:

- High presentation of researcher's voice – low presentation of participants' voices.
- High presentation of researcher's voice – high presentation of participants' voices.
- Low presentation of researcher's voice – low presentation of participants' voices.
- Low presentation of researcher's voice – high presentation of participants' voices.

Each of these choices has advantages and disadvantages which need to be considered in relation to the purposes of the study and the qualitative tradition within which it is located. As Pitney and Parker state:

> When explaining your study's emergent themes and findings, you must decide which participant quotes to use, how many quotes to use, and how much of your voice to share in the results section. These important considerations all relate to the issue of voice emphasis. In other words, which perspectives do you wish to highlight more, the participants' or your own? We believe that you must strike a balance between the two voices to present the results in a meaningful, compelling, and accurate manner.
>
> (Pitney & Parker, 2009: 102)

Besides participant quotations and researcher observations there are other ways to present findings in the results section. Wagstaff *et al.* (2012) provide a table at the start of their results section that provides the reader with a summary of key factors to emerge from their study. In the table, each key factor is named, a description of the findings in relation to this factor is given, and the applied implications of this are presented. This tactic is a useful way of crowding more in. For Wolcott (1990: 63–64), while qualitative research weds us to prose, we need to remind ourselves that charts, diagrams, maps, tables and photographs 'not only provide valuable supplements to printed text but can condense and expedite the presentation of supporting detail . . . Don't hesitate to explore alternative ways – and shapes – for displaying and summarising data using tables, figures, and maps'.

The use of such features will depend on intents and purposes of the researcher. For example, the narrative study by Sparkes, Perez-Samaniego, *et al.* (2012b) of the cancer experiences of an elite athlete and how these were shaped by the processes of narrative mapping and social comparisons relied extensively in its results section on direct quotes from the athlete which were supplemented by field observations to support emergent themes and describe key events. As such, a table or a diagram would not have added anything in their efforts to take the reader into the life-world of the athlete involved and how he made sense of his cancer experience. This is not to say that in their future work based on this case study that they will not include tables that summarise themes or use time-line diagrams.

Discussion or *Reflections*: This is normally the last section of a thesis or article, and for many qualitative studies it will also incorporate any *conclusions* that might be drawn from the research findings. This final section should not just be a 'summary' of what has already been said. For Silverman (2000) it needs to address the following questions:

- What is the relationship between the work done, the original research questions, previous work discussed in the literature review section and any new work appearing since the study began?
- If you were going to do the study again, is there anything you would do differently? If so – why? That is, what lessons can be learned from the way the study was conducted?
- What are the strengths and limitations of the study? What are the implications of these for the findings?
- What are the implications of the findings for policy and practice?
- What further research might follow from your findings, methods and concepts used?

In the discussion section of their paper on the *phenomenology* of gymnasts' lived experience, Post and Wrisberg (2012: 115–116) begin by linking their findings to the relevant literature in such statements as, 'the results appear to be consistent with Lang's bioinformational theory . . . The present findings also appear to be consistent with earlier research showing that elite athletes use imagery in a multisensory fashion'. They then identify how the current results also extend previous research by offering a more nuanced account of elite gymnasts' imagery. Next *noteworthy* findings that highlight this extension of thinking about imagery are focused upon, prior to the *unique* findings of the study being emphasised.

154

Having shown how their findings give a more complex picture of imagery than previous studies, Post and Wrisberg then proceed to reflect on the *theoretical implications* their findings have for future research in this area as well as the *practical implications* their work has for how coaches and sport psychologists can enhance gymnasts' imagery experiences. Finally, they consider two *limitations* of their findings before emphasising that despite each of these their study suggests that the imagery experience of athletes is a more complex phenomenon than previously depicted.

TRADITIONAL OR REALIST TALES

The structure we have provided above for representing qualitative work is traditional in its form and has been classed by Sparkes (2002a, 2008), following Van Maanen (1988), as a *realist tale*. This tale is characterised by the following conventions: *experiential author(ity)*; *the participant's point of view*; and *interpretive omnipotence*. Together, these conventions operate to foreground the voices of participants, allowing the reader to gain important insights into their perceptions of events. The orchestration and theoretical framing of these voices by a disembodied author are conventions that resonate with certain conventions of quantitative reporting, however, and this is a worry for some researchers. Of course, this does not make realist tales either good or bad. As Sparkes (2002a) acknowledges, realist tales, when well crafted, can provide compelling, detailed and complex depictions of a social world. Realist tales remain the dominant way of representing qualitative findings and will continue to make a major contribution to research into SEH.

The realist tale is not the only tale available to qualitative researchers in SEH. Against the backdrop of the *crisis of representation* that occurred in the 1980s, how we 'write' (explain, describe, index) the social were problematised (Denzin & Lincoln, 2000). Scholars came to realise that form and content are inseparable, so that the form of representation one uses has something to do with the form of understanding one secures. As Eisner (2008) emphasises, 'not only does knowledge come in different forms, the forms of its creation differ' (p. 5). In this sense, writing *is* a kind of analysis.

> I consider writing as a *method of inquiry*, a way of finding out about yourself and your topic. Although we usually think about writing as a mode of 'telling' about the social world, writing is

not just a mopping-up activity at the end of the research project. Writing is also a way of 'knowing' – a method of discovery and analysis. By writing in different ways, we discover new aspects of our topic and our relationship to it. Form and content are inseparable.

(Richardson, 2000: 923)

Experience is now taken to be *created* in the social text by the researcher, which means that the link between text and experience has become increasingly problematic. In view of this, creative analytical practices (CAP) have been developed in which authors move outside conventional social scientific writing forms.

In the wake of postmodernist – including poststructuralist, feminist, queer, and critical race theory – critiques of traditional qualitative writing practices, the sacrosanctity of social science writing conventions has been challenged. The ethnographic genre has been blurred, enlarged and altered with researchers writing in different formats for a variety of audiences.

(Richardson & St. Pierre, 2005: 962)

Against this backdrop, alternative forms of representation have been utilised by researchers in the social sciences (for example, Barone & Eisner, 2012; Gray & Sinding, 2002; Knowles & Cole, 2008; Saldaña, 2011b) which has had a direct influence on those working in SEH. Some of these will now be briefly considered.

CONFESSIONAL TALES

The confessional tale appeals to personalised authority and foregrounds the voice and concerns of the researcher about what happened during the fieldwork in a way that takes the reader behind the scenes of the 'cleaned up' methodological discussions so often provided in realist tales. The two main distinguishing characteristics of confessional tales are their highly personalised styles and their self-absorbed mandates. These fill the space in research that is left by the phenomenon of the 'missing researcher'. A reflexive stance (see Chapter 1) is adopted to explicitly problematise and demystify interviews, fieldwork or participant observation by revealing what actually happened in the research process from start to finish. The fieldwork odyssey, and the process and problems of coming to know, are the main focus rather than just the findings of the study. The ubiquitous, disembodied voice of the realist tale is replaced by the personal voice of the author announcing their presence: 'Here I am. This happened to me and this is how I felt, reacted and coped. Walk in my shoes for a while'.

An example of confessional tales can be found in the work of Douglas and Carless (2010). Alongside running a golf group programme for people experiencing severe and enduring mental health difficulties they also conducted an ethnographic research project to explore the socio-cultural dynamics of the programme. Having published several papers about their findings, they felt that something was still 'missing' from their existing writings when they returned to the transcripts and field notes.

> While our published analyses and interpretations were not wrong, they were seldom reflexive and they inadequately communicated the richness and complexity of what we had seen, heard and experienced. In essence, we found ourselves left with potentially important issues and insights that resisted expression through the realist tale genre we had relied upon.
>
> (Douglas & Carless, 2010: 337)

Douglas and Carless (2010) therefore constructed a confessional tale specifically because they wished to be an authorial presence in the text as opposed to a disembodied voice. By writing themselves into the research text they provided a degree of reflexivity that shed light on the ways factors concerning them as researchers might influence, for example, their interpretations and conclusions. They state: 'Our use here of a confessional tale can be seen as a methodological strategy which seeks to align with epistemologies that promote the creation of reflexive knowledge' (p. 338).

Another example of confessional tale can be found in the work of Fortune and Mair (2011). They reflect upon the impact of themselves as researchers in the production and interpretation of the data generated in their ethnographic study of a small sports club (curling) in rural Canada to investigate the role of such clubs as social and community spaces.

> Engaging in self-reflexivity and paying attention to our ethnographic presences enabled us to identify how our actions, assumptions, and motivations influenced the research. In other words, despite our commitment to adopting a consistent approach to

data collection and observation, the similarities and differences in terms of who we were before entering the club, and who we became while there, shaped how we engaged in the research.

(Fortune & Mair, 2011: 458)

As part of this self-reflexive process, Fortune and Mair draw extensively on their field notes to illustrate and problematise how their senses of self and positioning as a graduate assistant (Fortune) and an assistant professor (Mair) interacted to shape their interactions within the curling club, the kinds of data they collected, and the interpretations they consequently made. Specific attention is paid to role relationships, forms of participation, performing, personal issues (relating to background and experiences), and maintaining balance and distance. Their self-revealing text illustrates the problems that qualitative researchers have to grapple with on a regular basis, such as power, ethics, representation, voice, subjectivity and interpretation.

Set alongside realist representations of specific research projects, well-crafted confessional tales are of vital importance in generating a reflexive and critical stance towards both the process and the products of qualitative research. This genre of representation has a crucial role to play in highlighting the perils and pitfalls of the research experience, helping fellow inquirers learn from the private mistakes of others, and removing the inhibitions generated when novice researchers are fed solely on a diet of completed, methodologically sanitised, successful research projects. Given that confessional tales highlight fieldwork as a hermeneutic process, and raise a host of ethical and methodological questions about how we come to know about ourselves and others via our research activities, they have great pedagogical potential. As Van Maanen (1988) comments, 'the confessional becomes a self-reflective meditation on the nature of ethnographic understanding; the reader comes away with a deeper sense of the problems posed by the enterprise itself' (p. 92). On this basis alone, such tales make a positive contribution to our understanding of research into SEH.

AUTOETHNOGRAPHY

Autoethnography, or 'narratives of self' as it is sometimes called, is highly personalised, revealing writing in which researchers tell stories about their own lived experiences, relating the personal to the cultural. Ellis and Bochner (2000) define this genre of creative analytical practice as one that displays multiple layers of consciousness, as the autoethnographer gazes back and forth 'first through an ethnographic wide-angle lens, focusing outward on social and cultural aspects of their personal experience; then, they look inward, exposing a vulnerable self that is moved by and may move through, refract, and resist cultural interpretations' (p. 739). Autoethnographies vary in their emphasis on the research process (graphy), on culture (ethnos), and on self (auto). Likewise, Allen-Collinson (2012) states that, in general, 'autoethnography is a research approach which draws on the researcher's own personal lived experience, specifically in relation to the culture (and subcultures) of which s/he is a member' (p. 193). For her, given that the researcher, in her/his social interaction with others is the subject of the research, then the putative distinctions between the personal and the social, and between self and other, are necessarily blurred.

The conceptual framework for autoethnography, according to Chang (2008), is based on the following four assumptions:

1. Culture is a group-orientated concept by which the self is always connected with others;
2. The reading and writing of self-narrative provides a window through which the self and others can be examined and understood;
3. Telling one's story does not automatically result in the cultural understanding of self and others, which only grows out of in-depth cultural analysis and interpretation; and
4. Autoethnography is an excellent instructional tool to help not only social scientists but also practitioners gain profound understanding of self and other and function more effectively with others from diverse cultures. (Chang, 2008: 13)

A growing number of scholars have utilised autoethnography to explore various issues in SEH that include the following: the impact of sporting injury on the masculine self (Brown, Gilbourne & Claydon, 2009; Gilbourne, 2002; Sparkes, 1996, 2003a, 2003b); experiences of serious injury and the dynamics of the recovery process (Allen-Collinson, 2005, 2008); the dilemmas of a coach maintaining face in a difficult team setting (Jones, 2006); the sensory activity experienced by distance runners as they traverse their routine training routes (Hockey, 2006, 2013); the shared coach–athlete experience in competitive rowing with regard to power, consent and resistance (Purdy, Potrac, & Jones, 2008); identity construction and negotiation during a career as an elite woman golfer (Douglas, 2009); the construction, negotiation, and transformation of gendered identities through physical activity and sport (Krane, 2009); experiences of anorexia, excessive exercising and psychosis (Stone, 2009); the body in elite sport and the shaping of masculine identity (Drummond, 2010); the bodily experiences of an elite female swimmer as influenced by the regulatory practices of self and others (McMahon & Dinan-Thompson, 2011); identity development for young same-sex-attracted males in sport and physical education (Carless, 2012a); the embodiment of father–son relationships across generations via sporting practices (Sparkes, 2012); 'real life' ethical decision-making in the context of a symposium on sexual transgressions conducted during a professional conference on sport psychology (Dzikus *et al.*, 2012); and the problems, dilemmas and joys of working in academia and grappling with impact factors as an editor of an SEH journal (Smith, in press).

The exemplars cited above illustrate the point made by Allen-Collinson (2012) that in autoethnography, the roles of the researcher and participant coalesce so that the 'researcher's own experiences *qua* member of the social group and within social contexts are subject to analysis, in order to produce richly textured, often powerfully evocative accounts or even performances of lived experience' (p. 194). She notes that in such exemplars the autoethnographer occupies a dual, and often highly demanding role, both as a member of the social world under study and as a researcher of that same world. For Allen-Collinson, this demands of the autoethnographic researcher 'high levels of critical awareness and reflexivity and, many of us would add, self discipline . . . It can also initiate a challenging, intellectually demanding and emotionally painful voyage of self-investigation . . . [I]t is not for the faint-hearted' (p. 194).

Often, autoethnography as a genre is universally charged with being an act of self-indulgence, egocentrism and navel gazing, which, of course, it can be if poorly executed. This *universal* charge, as Allen-Collinson and Hockey (2005), and Sparkes (2000, 2002a, 2002b) point out, is however based on a number of misplaced assumptions about the purpose of autoethnography and the nature of the self–culture–society relationships that operate in and through them. To write individual experience is simultaneously to write social experience because if culture circulates through us all (and it does) then autoethnography is *always* connected to a world beyond the self. As such, well-crafted autoethnographies have the potential to challenge disembodied ways of knowing, and enhance empathetic forms of understanding by seeing our 'actual worlds' more clearly. Allen-Collinson (2012) makes the following observation:

> In inviting the reader to share the feeling and sensations, and to connect with the author's experience, autoethnographers often

160

write highly readable, insightful and thought-provoking work, vividly bringing alive sub/cultural experiences for those unfamiliar with the social terrain under study . . . Autoethnographic research offers, I would argue, a means of gaining rich and nuanced insights into personal lived experience and situating these within a wider socio-cultural context; insights which are unlikely to be accessible via more 'orthodox' research approaches.

(Allen-Collinson, 2012: 205–208)

Atkinson (2012) confirms that we can learn a great deal from autoethnographies about the particular social processes, experiences and realities involved in the unfolding of social life. He believes that in their 'opening up' of the personal they are also able to help readers better connect with academic arguments, theories and ideas. Consequently, well-crafted autoethnographies have the potential to add to our understanding of a range of phenomena in SEH and are worthy of development in the future.

POETIC REPRESENTATIONS

A poetic representation is where researchers transform their data into a poem-like composition, often using the exact words of the participants and arranging these to create a meaningful representation of the participant's lived experience. The process involves word reduction while at the same time illuminating the wholeness and interconnectedness of thoughts. Here, poetry is used as a vehicle to represent the data and the findings of a qualitative study to an audience in an evocative form.

Sparkes (2002a) suggests that constructing different poems about the same data can help a researcher to rethink the data and to work on additional ways to highlight these. Poetry offers a difference in forms of knowing as well as representing. Richardson (2000) likewise argues that 'settling words together in new configurations lets us see, and *feel* the world in new dimensions. Poetry is thus a *practical* and *powerful* method for analysing social worlds' (p. 933). Other advantages of poetic representations include the following:

- Writing up interviews as poems allows the speaker's pauses, repetitions, narrative strategies, rhythms, to be honoured. This may actually be a more *accurate* way of representing the speaker than the normal practice of quoting in prose snippets.

- Transforming data into poetry displays the role of the *prose trope* in constituting knowledge, and is a continual reminder to the reader or listener that the text has been artfully constructed. This dissolves any notion of separation between observer and observed.
- Poetic representations are able to create evocative and open-ended connections to the data for the researcher, reader and listener. This kind of creative analytical practice can touch both the cognitive and the sensory, recreate moments of experience, and show another person how it is to feel something, with an economy of words.
- People respond differently to poetry than they do to prose. When the dynamics of the reading or listening process are changed, the potential to elicit different responses arises.
- Poetic representations can provide the researcher, reader and listener with a different lens though which to view the same scenery, and thereby understand data, and themselves, in different and more complex ways.
- Given the volume of data generated by interviews, poetic representations can communicate the findings of a study in a condensed form with an economy of words.

The potential benefits for both the author and the reader of poetic representation are evident in the work of those who have chosen to use this genre in SEH (for example, see Carless, 2012b; Carless & Douglas, 2009a; Chawansky, 2011; Gilbourne, 2011; Sparkes, 2012; Sparkes, Nilges, Swan & Dowling, 2003; and Sparkes & Douglas, 2007). For example, Fitzpatrick (2012) spent over 300 hours in health and physical education classes with high school students in New Zealand as part of her critical ethnographic study that focused on young people's perspectives of health, physical education and schooling. She suggests that representing some of her findings in poetic form provides a rich, evocative and aesthetic means of communicating her data to others which, in turn, enhances her critical ethnographic work in ways that bring the personal and the political together. Importantly, Fitzpatrick emphasises that transforming her data into poetry gave her a different way to 'look' at the site of her research and to get inside and appreciate the cultural diversity therein.

Drawing on a larger study that sought to better understand women's experiences as recruited athletes within the US intercollegiate sports system, Chawansky (2011) utilised interview data with seven women recruited to play Division One basketball, to construct a series of poems

162

called *Lust, Euphoria, Fear, Disgust, The Truth*, and *The Finale*. Discussing her rationale for using poetic representations, Chawansky notes the limitations of existing academic research on the topic of recruitment and how this leaves us with little understanding of what it means for women to be recruited, what methods are used to recruit women athletes, and how women athletes make sense of their recruiting experiences. Here poems, therefore, seek to engage some of the unanswered questions surrounding athletic recruiting and to attend to the emotional responses that accompany them:

> What does it mean to be wanted? To be watched? To be wooed by a university and then dropped? What changes as one transitions from recruit to university athlete/recruiter? Finally, what do we still need to know about recruiting, and how can we best represent these stories?
>
> (Chawansky, 2011: 5)

Sparkes and Douglas (2007) constructed a poetic representation to analyse and communicate the experiences of one participant, named Leanne, involved in a larger interview-based study that explored the multiple meanings of motivation over time for a group of seven elite, female, golf professionals. Importantly, they take the reader through the process by which the data from interviews with Leanne (35 pages of single spaced script) were transformed into a sequence of four poetic representations called *My Dad, The Pressure, Playing The Tour*, and *Coming To My Senses*. For example, using excerpts from interview transcripts they illustrate how, where possible, only the words of Leanne and the order they were spoken in were used in order to give a sense of the narrative flow of her speech and convey some of the meanings she attached to specific events. During multiple listenings to the interviews, Douglas paid careful attention to the stresses and accents Leanne placed on certain words and phrases along with her repetitions and how these formed key themes in her story. Leanne continually returned to the powerful influence of her father who motivated her to take up golf and succeed in this sport. The contradictions and unhappiness that Leanne experienced in playing golf tours, along with her gradual realisation that she could make her own decisions and retire prematurely if she wanted to were also recurrent themes in the interviews. Given the importance of these key themes in Leanne's life, each was used as a framing device for the construction of a poetic representation.

Reflecting on the reactions of various audiences to the poetic representations, which included Leanne herself, university undergraduate students, and delegates at an international conference. Sparkes and Douglas (2007) note how these have raised awareness in relation to a number of key theoretical and practical issues. These include the following: allowing the audience to see and analyse familiar sporting situations in new and challenging ways; evoking a range of responses; encouraging a reflexive stance toward self and others; allowing for a more holistic understanding of motivation and mental well-being in different contexts; and having a direct impact on policy changes. They suggest, therefore, that much might be gained from researchers in SEH creating poetic representations from in-depth interviews and other data from the field.

ETHNODRAMA/THEATRE

Performing data is an immensely powerful way of presenting research. Speaking of *performance ethnography* as an emerging creative analytic practice, Atkinson (2012) notes how, having spent time in the field, the ethnographer, generally in conjunction with key informants from the group under study, writes and produces a dramatic play, vignette or short film representing the culture. By using the theatre or the screen as a place of representation, 'performance ethnography transforms them from a place of entertainment to a venue for participatory action research that extends beyond the performance itself' (p. 31). As a forum for cultural exchange, Atkinson argues that the power of performance ethnography lies in its 'potential for illumination and engagement of involved researchers, participants and audience' (p. 32).

One type of performance ethnography is *ethnodrama*. For Mienczakowski and Moore (2008) ethnodrama is a method and methodology that combine 'qualitative research processes with action research, grounded theory, and narrative to provide data from which a script can be written that, in turn, becomes the basis of health theatre' (p. 451). Ethnodrama relies upon the voices, lived experiences and beliefs of its participants to inform its content, shape and intent. Importantly, Mienczakowski and Moore argue that performed data have an 'empathetic power and dimension often lacking in standard qualitative research narratives' (p. 451).

Another type of performance ethnography is *ethnotheatre*. In making an important distinction between *ethnodrama* and *ethnotheatre*, Saldaña

(2011b) notes that both are rooted in non-fictional, researched reality before offering the following definitions.

> *Ethnotheatre*, a word joining *ethnography* and *theatre*, employs the traditional craft and artistic techniques of theatre or media production to mount for an audience a live or mediated performance event of research participants' experiences and/or the researchers' interpretations of data. The goal is to investigate a particular facet of the human condition for purposes of adapting those observations and insights into a performance medium. This investigation is preparatory fieldwork for theatrical production work.

> An *ethnodrama*, a word joining *ethnography* and *drama*, is a written play script consisting of dramatized, significant selections of narrative collected from interview transcripts, participant observation field notes, journal entries, personal memories/ experiences, and/or print and media artifacts such as diaries, blogs, e-mail correspondence, television broadcasts, newspaper articles, court proceedings, and historic documents. In some cases production companies can work improvisationally and collaboratively to devise original and interpretive texts based on authentic sources. Simply put, this is dramatizing data.
>
> (Saldaña, 2011b: 13)

Researchers might choose an ethnodramatic play script and its ethnotheatrical production to represent their findings, Saldaña (2011b) suggests, because they have determined that these art forms are the most appropriate and effective modalities for communicating their observations of cultural, social, or personal life. Many audience members who attend an effective theatre production, even if the play is fictional, testify afterward that the live performance event made the phenomena focused upon seem more 'real.' He argues that if this art form has the ability and the power to heighten the representation and presentation of social life, 'and if our research goal with a particular fieldwork project is to capture and document the stark realities of the people we talked to and observed, then the medium of theatre seems the most compatible choice for sharing our findings and insights' (p. 15). Thus, this kind of creative analytical practice is a very effective form of *knowledge translation*.

Besides making phenomena seem more 'real', further reasons why qualitative researchers in SEH might transform their data and analysis into ethnodrama/theatre include the following:

- It captures the lived experiences of participants in the study (including the researcher–author) in ways that remain true(r) to those experiences. More conventional forms of reporting are often not as capable of accomplishing this task.
- It can give voice to what is unspoken.
- It presents research findings in a thought-provoking, engaging and accessible manner to wider and diverse audiences beyond the academy that engages them both cognitively and emotionally. The research can, therefore, have wide and significant impact.
- It can be an innovative way to challenge readers and audiences about the dominant stereotypes and myths they hold concerning both the lived realities of specific groups and those who work with them.
- It allows researchers to understand and analyse their data in a very different way.
- It allows researchers, should they decide to become an actor in the drama, to connect to the lived reality of their participants in new and richer ways. That is, through their whole bodies as they feel the data in their bones and flesh.

A number of researchers in SEH have opted to transform their data into ethnodrama/theatre. For example, drawing on data generated from an ethnographically-informed study that explored the exposure and effect of culture in relation to body practices with adolescent swimmers, McMahon, Penney and Dinan-Thompson (2012) chose to represent their findings as what Saldaña (2011b) would describe as an ethnodrama. That is, they transformed the stories told by the participants about their body practices into what they describe as a 'theatrical format', presenting a play in the form of two acts. Each act is made up of a series of stories (vignettes), where a story from the life of each of the three main actors (participants) is told though a theatrical and ethnographic lens. In reflecting on their reasons for choosing such an approach, McMahon and her colleagues make the following points:

> The acts are consciously staged as the actors' own production, seeking to maximise their authoritative voices . . . The vignettes within each act have a number of distinguishing features. They capture language occurring from multiple dimensions, the feelings, thoughts, tensions and inner monologue of participants, with the intention of provoking reader emotion. Each vignette seeks to provide new insights into the life of the swimmer with

the use of vernacular language, provoking dramatic potential. The main force, focus and tension of each vignette are created though character dialogue . . . The reader is invited into their personal story and should be able to feel empathy with the actors, relating to, but not having to endure their experience.

(McMahon et al., 2012: 186)

In 2000, based on her life history interviews with eight physical educators who self-identified as 'queer', 'lesbian' and 'gay' physical education teachers, Sykes, in collaboration with two actors/drama educators (Chapman and Swedberg), produced what she called a 'performed ethnography'. Fitting with Saldaña's (2011b) notion of ethnotheatre, this twenty-five minute performance called *Wearing the Secret Out* deals with issues such as coming out, homophobic violence and same-sex desire in physical education.

Reflecting on the process of creating and performing this performed ethnography Sykes, Chapman and Swedberg (2006) note that pedagogically it was designed to generate incomplete and multiple meanings. Thus, the performance did not claim that students in the audience would 'learn' how to teach in less homophobic or heterosexist ways. Rather, the performance was intended to address the 'multiple whos' in the audience so as to create 'multiple possibilities for identification and dis-identification for each member of the audience. Ultimately this performed ethnography gives students an obligation to make their own meanings about how to approach anti-homophobic teaching' (p. 189). *Wearing The Secret Out* has been performed live or shown as a video to a wide range of audiences and at a variety of academic conferences specialising in physical education and sport. Sykes and her colleagues note the range of embodied reactions from audience members that confirms, for them, the value of performance ethnography as a mode of representation.

According to Sparkes (2002a), virtually any qualitatively orientated study, focusing on participants' own telling of their life situations, can provide a foundation for later dramatic work – although the parameters of the study may put limits on what the drama can subsequently address. As Sparkes (2002a) and Gray and Sinding (2002) emphasise, however, the creation of a drama in itself in no way ensures broader access to social science research, nor does it ensure that researchers will make a difference in the world. If the ethnodrama/theatre is done *badly*, then none of its potential will be realised. In fact, it might turn people away from engaging with the important issues the data raised in the studies mentioned. Therefore, given the lack of knowledge and skill that most researchers in SEH are likely to have in drama or theatre, it is appropriate to seek guidance, support and collaboration with those who have specific expertise in the performing arts as part of this venture.

One does not have to be a trained theatre artist to write ethnodrama and produce ethnotheatre. However, as Saldaña (2011b) suggests, *collaborative ventures* between social scientists and theatre practitioners are more likely to produce higher quality research-based work on stage. The reasons why are made evident in his following statement:

> *A play is not a journal article.* They are two completely different genres of writing, each with its own distinctive traditions, elements, and styles. I am usually the kind of mentor who encourages people to find their own creative direction, but I will be quite unwavering on this point: don't even *think* about including footnotes or citations of the relevant literature in your play script. A play is not a journal article; you do not need references after the play is over. If the play can't speak for itself, then you either need to rewrite the script till it does, or find a more accommodating literary genre to say what you have to say. You may also be in trouble if you envision your stage setting to include a lectern, or if the action is set in a university classroom or faculty office. *A play is not a journal article. So stop thinking like a social scientist and start thinking like an artist.*
> (Saldaña, 2011b: 36–37, emphasis in original)

The move towards a performance medium requires that researchers extend themselves well beyond the roles that they have acquired expertise in and feel secure with. With regard to performing data to a live audience, Bagley (2009) notes how it requires the researcher to be culturally and politically sensitive:

> The relational positioning of the researcher towards content (what is selected to be performed), art form (the maintenance of the integrity of the genre), artists (who is selected and their role), audience (to whom we perform), interviewees (how much and what is revealed), and staging of the performance (how is it structured to communicate meaning) are all integral to the enactment

of a meaningful performative endeavour and collectively speak to the performance ethic.

(Bagley, 2009: 285)

With regard to performance ethics, drawing on their own experiences of producing ethnodrama/theatre, Mienczakowski and Moore (2008) offer some interesting reflections on the notions of responsibility in performing data. They recommend that prior to any performance, that attempts are made to anticipate any ethical and moral dilemmas that may arise with regard, for example, the impact on audience members (who may include members of the vulnerable groups on which the performance is based), the researchers who provided the data, and the actors themselves. As Mienczakowski and Moore note, there is a need to take account of a range of unwanted and unintended outcomes that may arise directly through unforeseen emotional responses to the performance. For them, 'Remaining true to the rich data comes with ethical dilemmas . . . With these potential risks come a social responsibility for the care of our informants and participants' (pp. 454–455).

As described above, there are many benefits for researchers in SEH in transforming qualitative data into ethnodrama/theatre. That said, there are also risks involved that the researcher needs to be aware of before they engage with this genre. Given the possibilities and risks involved we would suggest that the best way forward is the development of mutually beneficial and respectful collaborations with those who have expertise in the domains of drama and theatre and those who inhabit the domains of SEH.

ETHNOGRAPHIC NONFICTIONS

A number of scholars have made the case for using what has variously been called literary fiction or creative nonfiction, as a productive, valuable and necessary mode of expression in certain circumstances for communicating scholarship and research findings (Banks, 2008; Barone, 2008; Caulley, 2008; Denison & Markula, 2003; Smith, 2013b; Sparkes, 2002a, 2002c, 2007; Watson, 2011). As a way of representing ethnographic data, Angrosino (2007) notes the following:

> *Fiction* is any literary form in which the setting and people who are studied in that setting are represented fictionally (e.g.

use of composite characters, setting characters in hypothetical events, attributing revelatory interior monologues to people when the researcher could not possibly have heard the original discourse). Fiction is sometimes employed for ethical reasons (the better to disguise the identities of people who might be compromised if they were too readily identified by conventionally 'objective' writing), sometimes to make a better link between the experiences of the study community and more universal concerns.

(Angrosino, 2007: 80–81)

Angrosino (2007: 81) emphasises that when researchers speak of fictional representations of ethnographic data, this does *not* mean that they are talking about making things up and disguising them as facts. For him, 'Fictional representation merely refers to the use of the techniques of literary fiction, rather than the conventions of academic prose, to tell a story; by general consensus, works of ethnographic fiction are clearly labelled as such'. This view is supported by Banks (2008: 162) who states that when fictions are created to share a research experience with readers, 'it is necessary for them to declare their fictional nature'.

Leaving aside the complex debates and challenges regarding the traditional fact/fiction dualism and the blurring of boundaries due to the use of 'fiction' as a representational form, many qualitative researchers appear more comfortable associating their work with the terms 'literary nonfiction' or 'creative nonfiction'. According to Sparkes (2002a, 2002b), the use of these terms makes it clear to the reader that their stories are based on 'real' events and people and that the researcher was 'there' in the action as a participant observer, or has generated data by other methods in a systematic manner. Thus, an ethnographic creative nonfiction is a type of creative analytic practice that is grounded in research findings and draws on literary techniques to produce a story. The story produced is 'real' and not wholly 'imagined'. It is fictional in form but factual in content. It tells a story using facts and is deeply committed to the 'truth', but uses many of the techniques of fiction for its emotional vibrancy and compelling qualities. As Barone (2000) notes:

But for an educational portrait to have real value, it is essential that authors use as their material the actual, particular, specific phenomena confronted in the research setting . . . Unlike the

170

artist, the evaluator is therefore not entirely free to disregard literal 'truth'. If such an educational portrait is to be convincing, especially to those familiar with the particular research scene, then not least of its virtues must be accuracy. Its characters and setting must be actual, not virtual. Their descriptions should consist of a host of personality indicators, of physical attributes and characteristics of human behavior, in actual incidents, recorded comments, and so on.

(Barone, 2000: 24–25)

Readers of creative nonfiction can presume that the events actually happened but that the factual evidence is being shaped and dramatised using fictional techniques that include evocative and metaphoric language techniques (for example, vernacular language; composite characters; inner dialogue; flashbacks and flash forwards; tone shifts and so on) to provide a forceful, coherent rendering of events that appeals to aesthetic criteria (among others) rather than simply being 'objectively' and 'factually' reported via 'thin' descriptions. The reader is invited to vicariously participate in the events described and to feel the immediacy of the experiences of those involved. Using the scenic method, the researcher *shows* rather than *tells*.

A number of scholars within SEH have opted to use creative nonfiction as a way of representing their findings. For example, Carless and Sparkes (2008), having conducted semi-structured interviews with three men with serious mental illness (SMI) about their experiences of physical activity, opted to represent their findings in the form of three creative nonfiction short stories. They made this choice for a number of reasons:

- They wanted to invite diverse interpretations, rather than narrow and closed interpretations of their findings, by taking the reader into the experiential world of SMI and allowing them to make sense of it from their own unique vantage point (for example, a person living with severe mental illness, a psychiatric nurse, a psychiatrist, a health professional, or an exercise and sport psychologist).
- Given that much of the existing mental health literature is characterised by a focus on the deficiencies, deficits and problems of mental illness, they wanted to counterbalance this tendency towards negative outcomes and expectations by providing positive stories of living with SMI that suggest a vision of possibilities of what can be achieved by those with this sort of illness.

- Given that historically, people with SMI have been excluded from professional dialogue and their voices not heard as members of a silenced and marginalised population, the story form was chosen because it provided a direct focus on the voices of those who experience SMI.
- Given the challenges that SMI presents for service users, family members, and carers, the availability of SMI stories offers the possibility of becoming part of a collective story that generates a sense of solidarity connecting people with SMI together in ways that challenge the feelings of isolation that often prevail.
- Given that people with SMI are one of the most stigmatised sections of society resulting primarily from a lack of understanding of what it is like to live with this kind of illness, stories of such lives make available accessible and alternative perspectives that can challenge misplaced views by illustrating what people with SMI have in common with others in society so that empathetic bonds across difference can be created.

Fictional approaches, Douglas and Carless (2009) suggest, are useful for exploring taboo, silenced and 'dangerous' issues that are often excluded from research and practice in elite and professional sport. Based on a series of interviews and conversations with a successful professional woman golfer, Douglas and Carless present what they term as an 'ethnographic fiction' that explores the issue of sexual harassment and abuse in sport by unfolding a story about events leading up to the rape of this golfer by a caddie whist on tour. The fictional approach was chosen by them because, in this instance, it offers a cloak of anonymity which is an ethical necessity given the experiences recounted in the story. Besides this, Douglas and Carless, having previously utilised a realist telling, felt that this genre was not suitable to represent the experiences they had been given access to as witnesses of another's life story.

> We had witnessed a silenced story that needed to be told, one that was 'unrecognised or suppressed.' We felt uncomfortable pathologising the teller, recounting her stories as 'detached' experts'. Instead we sought to put her experiences in context in a way that might lead others to stand with her, understand her difficulties, and appreciate their own role in events of this type. Fictional writing offered us the best chance of achieving this aim . . . In this regard, the creation of fiction is one way a writer/

researcher deepens her knowledge of human behaviour through stretching the limits of her imaginary visions. We document, in our minds, the minute details of our characters, their movements and glances, as well as what they feel, hear, see, touch and imagine when we recreate them in order that others can see.

(Douglas & Carless, 2009: 316)

More recently, Waldron, Lynn and Krane (2011) examined 'hazing' activities in high school sport that are intended to humiliate, degrade and abuse new team members with the presumed outcome of enhancing team bonding. They conducted focus group interviews with nine former high-school athletes to explore their experiences of hazing and then subjected the data to a narrative analysis. Following this, based on the data from these male athletes, they used 'creative nonfiction' techniques to compose three stories, in the form of monologues. Two of these focused on 'being hazed' and the other on 'enacting hazing'. In justifying their genre choice Waldron and her colleagues pointed out that the story form enabled them to provide thick descriptions of the lived hazing experiences as well as a consideration of why they occurred and the consequences of the events.

Providing a complete story, via a monologue, presents the text with concrete details and in a complete manner . . . [T]he monologues meld the voices of all the athletes in the focus groups; that is, much of the text is direct quotes from the interviews. Our goal of such a format is for these stories to resonate with readers and create deeper understanding of the psychological and emotional components of these athletes' experiences.

(Waldron *et al.*, 2011: 115)

The exemplars of creative nonfiction and storied forms of communication provided above suggest that this approach has much to offer researchers in SEH. This is particularly so in terms of their *pedagogical* potential. Strong evidence for this potential is provided by Douglas and Carless (2008) (see also Smith, 2013b) who conducted a series of professional development seminars for golf coaches in which they presented a number of previously published stories (and poetic representations) that explored the experiences of female professional tournament golfers. Feedback from the coaches about their reactions to each of the stories was collected via the use of questionnaires and a focus group. Following each seminar a debriefing session was held during which time Douglas and Carless recorded further reactions, thoughts and observations in their reflexive diaries about the coaches' reactions. An analysis of the feedback from the coaches found that they responded in three different ways that involved *questioning, summarising* and *incorporating* the story. These three response styles, Douglas and Carless suggest, provide evidence that the stories stimulated a degree of reflection and critical thinking about holistic issues such as athlete well-being and career progression. These do so by provide a catalyst for coaches to

> explore their own subjective, moral and ethical beliefs in a supportive environment which more closely aligns with the dynamic nature of their work. This process is necessary if coaches are to find ethically and morally informed resolutions to the many complex issues that arise in high-performance sport.
>
> (p. 46)

Adopting a similar approach, Douglas and Carless (2009) analyse the responses and reactions of university students to their story about sexual abuse in elite professional sport. The responses indicate that the students found the story to be a powerfully emotive and authentic account that stimulates them to incorporate the story within their own life and express feelings of empathy with the story teller via a process of identification with the events, motives and orientations of the characters involved. Instrumental to this process of active reflection is the provision of space for the voices and perspectives of 'others' to be heard and acknowledged in ways that destabilises students' previously held assumptions about gender, sexuality and power in sport and raises numerous ethical issues for consideration. Douglas and Carless conclude that stories like the one they constructed have an important role to play in stimulating reflective practice in SEH settings.

Despite the potential benefits of using stories of a nonfictional kind within SEH settings it needs to be recognised that many researchers react very negatively when the word 'fiction' is linked in any way to the word 'research'. As Banks (2008) states, 'Fiction *per se*, however, still struggles for legitimacy in the academy as scholarly writing' (p. 160). Echoing this, Barone (2008) notes that in Western culture, fiction continues to be associated with the fantastic, and, as such, remains a no-no mode of expression, is off-limits in conventional academic discourse, reviled as tainted,

174

and dismissed as an academic half-breed! Despite all this, a small but growing number of scholars, in the social sciences in general and within SEH in particular, are choosing to utilise fictional forms to represent their findings, and they are getting published in international peer-reviewed journals. Most importantly of all, this genre is proving to be very useful for disseminating research findings to diverse audiences in an engaging, understandable and 'high impact' fashion (Smith, 2013b).

MUSICAL PERFORMANCE

Bresler (2008) explores the ways in which the various musical processes of listening, performing, composing and improvising can inform the processes of social science research in terms of relationships to participants, co-researchers, plus the audience of research and meaning making and conceptualisations in observations, data analysis and writing.

> Musical experiences can help reveal important dimensions of qualitative inquiry that have not been explored. Where sight gives us physical entities, the heard world is phenomenologically evanescent, relentlessly moving, ever changing. Involvement in music as creators, performers, and listeners requires that we engage in the evanescent aspects of world, cultivating sensibilities that apply to ways of doing as well as ways of *becoming*. These are the very same sensibilities that are needed for researches of human sciences.
>
> (Bresler, 2008: 226)

Music, according to Bresler (2008), connects to qualitative research via three specific themes: systematic improvisation, disciplined empathy, and embodiment. Regarding the latter she notes that sound penetrates us, and engages us on a bodily level in ways that are fundamentally different than the visual and so have an important part to play in the quest of qualitative research to illuminate and communicate lived experiences. As Bresler concludes, 'The fluidity of sound and music sensitizes us to the ephemeral, to the ebb and flow of lived and researched experience. Therein lie lessons from music' (p. 234).

In SEH, these lessons from music are beginning to be explored. For example, Carless and Douglas (2008) gathered data from interviews and field observations to explore the physical activity experiences of older women living in Cornwall in the UK. Having analysed their data in various ways, they felt that the use of standard scientific and realist tales would not be up to the task of dealing with the complexities they encountered in the study. Therefore, they created a 30-minute performance piece entitled *Across the Tamar* which incorporates songs, poems and stories stemming from the research. Speaking of their journey towards becoming what they call 'performative social science researchers' that culminated in them collaborating to produce *Across the Tamar*, Carless and Douglas (2010b) note that their performances to a range of audiences, including academics, and the participants in the original study and other gatherings of older people, have been greeted with more enthusiasm, passion and emotion than any other research that they had been involved with to date.

According to Carless and Douglas (2009b), the complex and necessarily unpredictable process of songwriting is an embodied practice that can be the source or stimulus for new understandings. Driven by a desire for connection combined with the opportunity to discover through writing, they see song-writing as a meaning-making process in which new knowledge and understanding can be accessed or created. Furthermore, 'it can also be an effective way to help bring embodied meaning to the creative process' (p. 35). This point is developed further by Carless and Douglas (2011) in their consideration of how songwriting can act as an alternative way both to acquire knowledge and communicate insights into the social world. They explore audience responses to their performance pieces *Across the Tamar* and *Under One Roof*. The latter is a 35-minute performance based on ethnographic research commissioned by the Addiction Recovery Agency into the lives and needs of people aged 50 or over who live in an urban supported housing scheme (Carless & Douglas, 2010).

Prior to the performances, Carless and Douglas (2011) distributed feedback sheets to audience members which asked them a series of open-ended questions designed to elicit their responses to the performances and what (if anything) they had learned through the performance. At the end of each performance they also engaged in a 30-minute informal discussion to access the audience's responses and reactions to the performance. During these public sessions Douglas took notes of the issues raised and the comments offered. Their analysis of audience feedback condensed around five interrelated themes. These were engagement and impact, stimulating emotional responses, supporting embodied knowing and triggering personal

176

reflection and local knowledge. For Carless and Douglas the evidence contained within these themes and their interactions suggest that songs can make an important, and perhaps unique, contribution to knowledge creation and communication and, as another creative analytical practice, it is worthy of serious consideration by qualitative researchers.

Utilising music as a way of understanding and analysing data, and communicating our findings to others, is not a task to be taken lightly. It is a process of engagement and development that comes with its own risks. Reflecting on her own journey into songwriting, Douglas (2012: 529) notes, 'It seems that for many scholars creating and singing song, as a way of understanding and representing their work, is an inaccessible mode of inquiry'. She recognises that for some, the move from scientific texts to songs is a big step, particularly for those individuals who normally separate their 'academic' selves from their 'creative and artistic' selves. As part of her own transition, Douglas points out that it required her to think through where her desire to write a song came from, 'to consider why I wanted to write a song from my research. What purpose would it bring? What would it contribute that couldn't be learned or presented in another way? What new or alternative insights would it allow?' (p. 527). This said, Douglas challenges the often-held view that one must be able to sing competently, write music and play an instrument before engaging in the song writing process. While acknowledging that there is some truth in the belief that in order to produce a 'professional performance' that includes songs, some degree of competency is necessary, her own personal experiences show that song-writing moments can draw on different levels of competencies, maturity, and skill that will change over time and in relation to an active engagement with others who do have expertise in a given genre.

SUMMARY

In this chapter we first outlined a traditional and well-respected structure for representing the findings of qualitative research. Following this, we then explored a variety of different arts-informed creative analytical practices, or genres, that can be called upon by qualitative researchers in SEH to both analyse and represent their findings in different ways. We acknowledged that each genre can offer a variety of things regarding the ways we come to understand the social world. We also noted that each was not without its problems and that informed choices need to be made about when, where, and if they are utilised.

Our intention has been to give a flavour of how the arts and qualitative inquiry are fusing together in ways that are opening up possibilities for alternative perspectives, modes, media, and genres through which to understand and represent the human condition. This sentiment is echoed by Bagley and Castro-Salazar (2012) who offer the following summary of the methodological possibilities of critical arts-based research as a genre within the qualitative paradigm:

> To engage with the emotional, sensual, and kinaesthetic complexity of everyday lived experiences; to challenge dominant cultural norms, beliefs and values; and to uncover, recover and portray research to audiences in new ways. In so doing, we contend, critical arts-based research in education is able to politically move subjects, performers, audience and researchers into new cultural spaces of understanding, resistance and hope.
>
> (Bagley & Castro-Salazar, 2012: 19)

Given the possibilities now available, we hope that, having become competent in crafting the realist tale, some researchers, when the moment is right, and with appropriate support, will take up the challenge of experimenting with other genres of representation as alternative ways to analyse, know, and communicate with others about the multiple lived realities of those who inhabit the world of SEH.

CHAPTER 7

JUDGING THE QUALITY OF QUALITATIVE RESEARCH

Judgments of quality in quantitative research revolve around issues of objectivity, reliability, generalisability and validity. Given that qualitative research is different then, as Tracy (2010) comments, applying these traditional criteria is illegitimate, 'akin to Catholic questions directed to a Methodist audience' (p. 838). How then should the quality of qualitative research be judged?

The most popular approach in SEH is founded on the work of Lincoln and Guba (1985) and Guba and Lincoln (1989). They acknowledged that qualitative research was based on a different ontology and epistemology than quantitative research, and then developed *parallel* criteria for judging its goodness that are ostensibly meaningful and relevant to qualitative work. In place of the conventional criteria of internal validity, external validity, reliability and objectivity they proposed the following parallel criteria: *credibility, transferability, dependability* and *confirmability*. Taken together these constitute the *trustworthiness* criteria that can be used to judge the 'quality' of qualitative research studies. These criteria currently constitute the gold standard in qualitative work in SEH.

The parallel perspective on criteria has not gone unquestioned. It is important to recognise that notions of generalisability, reliability and validity, and judgment criteria in general, are contested and debated issues with various groups and traditions within qualitative research adopting different positions towards them. This chapter aims to give a flavour of these debates and a sense of the different positions available so that the reader can make an informed choice about where they stand on key issues, what kind of strategies they might adopt to achieve certain criteria in relation to their research, and so feel confident to defend their work in the public domain. As Wolcott (1995) argues, qualitative researchers need to understand what these debates are about in terms of the principles involved and *have* a position. They do not, however, have to resolve these debates.

RELIABILITY

From a quantitative perspective, reliability is one of the most important features in determining a psychometrically sound research instrument, and refers to the consistency, repetition and reproducability of measures. Pitney and Parker (2009) acknowledge that this notion of reliability does not fit in with the assumptions of the qualitative enterprise. For them, because qualitative researchers do not rely on measurements and do not perform trials of activities or conduct the same interview twice, 'they do not need to worry about whether data can be reproduced' (p. 62). For Wolcott (1995), reliability remains beyond the pale for research based on observation in natural settings.

> In order to achieve reliability in that technical sense, a researcher has to manipulate conditions so that replicability can be assessed. Ordinarily, fieldworkers do not try to make things happen at all, but whatever the circumstances, we cannot *make* them happen twice. When something does happen more than once, we do not for a minute insist that this repetition is exact.
>
> (Wolcott, 1995: 167)

In other words, we cannot step into the same stream twice! Qualitative researchers, therefore, need to recognise the circumstances that render reliability as less than relevant to their concerns. They do not need to apologise for this, though. While reliability is a valuable quality in laboratory, medical and product safety research, and is valuable in *some* social science operations, a misplaced concern for this issue results in severe limits being placed on what the qualitative enterprise should include. Accordingly, Wolcott (1995) suggests, that qualitative researchers need not address reliability at all in their work 'except to make sure that our audiences understand why it is not an appropriate measure for evaluating fieldwork' (p. 168).

Qualitative researchers who *are* concerned with reliability have dealt with it in the form of *dependability*. For Guba and Lincoln (1989), 'dependability is parallel to the conventional criterion of reliability, in that it is concerned with the stability of the data over time' (p. 242). They recognise that given the nature of qualitative research that reliability, in a quantitative sense, is an impossibility. For them, however, as part of establishing the trustworthiness of their work, researchers can achieve the parallel notion of dependability by providing a dependability audit and including an audit trail. These strategies are used to

180

convince the consumer of the inquiry that the process is logical, traceable and documented.

The dependability and inquiry audit is a procedure based on the metaphor (and actual process) of the fiscal audit in which two kinds of issues are explored. These are: to what extent is the process an established, trackable and documentable process; and to what extent are various data in the book-keeping system actually confirmable. For a study to be judged as dependable, it must be consistent and accurate. It is the responsibility of researchers to demonstate this by providing an audit trail in which they give detailed descriptions of the path of their research and decision-making processes so that the reader can inspect these. With this audit trail in place, readers are then able to carry out an inquiry or dependability audit in which they follow the path of the research and make their own judgement about its dependability.

OBJECTIVITY

Closely linked to Lincoln and Guba (1985) and Guba and Lincoln's (1989) notion of dependability is *confirmability*. Confirmability is the parallel to the conventional criterion of *objectivity*. It is concerned with assuring that the data, interpretations and outcomes of inquiries are rooted in the contexts and persons *apart* from researchers so that the results of the inquiry are not the outcome of the biases and 'rampant' subjectivity of researchers or are simply based on figments of their imagination. The technique they suggest to achieve this criterion involves uncovering the decision-making trail of the researcher and making it available for public judgment. This is known as the *confirmability audit*.

> Unlike the conventional paradigm, which roots its assurances of objectivity in method . . . [t]he constructivist paradigm's assurances of integrity of the findings are rooted in the data themselves. This means that data (constructions, assertions, facts, and so on) can be tracked to their sources, and that the logic used to assemble the interpretations into structurally coherent and corroborating wholes is both explicit and implicit in the narrative of the case study. Thus, both the 'raw products' and the 'processes used to compress them', are available to be inspected and confirmed by outside reviewers of the study.
>
> (Guba & Lincoln, 1989: 243)

Given their core assumptions, qualitative researchers realise the futility of attempting to achieve objectivity. They do seek, however, to be *reflexive* about their work and to show that the data they produced can be traced back to its origins and that they have made informed, strategic and principled methodological decisions along with fair and balanced interpretations (see Chapter 1). According to Wolcott (1995) such reflexivity involves a *disciplined subjectivity*. For him, *good* bias in research is unavoidable and necessary. By lending a focus it is essential to the performance of any research. He notes, 'in the total absence of bias, a researcher would be unable even to leave the office to set off in the direction of a potential research site' (p. 165). In contrast, *bad* bias is a matter of excess.

> In the case of qualitative research, bias becomes excessive to whatever extent it exerts undue influence on the consequences of the inquiry. In the extreme, conclusions may be foreordained without investigation of any kind. To guard against this is not to deny bias or pretend to suppress it, but to recognise it and harness it. Bias should stimulate inquiry without interfering with the investigation. That surely requires art. The critical step is to understand that *bias itself is not the problem*. One's purposes and assumptions need to be made explicit and used judiciously to give meaning and focus to the study.
>
> (Wolcott, 1995: 165)

Concerns over bias, therefore, require that researchers identify the perspectives they bring to their studies as insiders and/or as outsiders and to anticipate how these may affect how they analyse, interpret and report the findings. Without this reflexive self-awareness the true foe of the qualitative researcher, *prejudice*, can creep in and allow judgments to form without an explicit basis. Therefore, as Wolcott (1995) recommends 'covet your biases, display them openly, and ponder how they can help you formulate both the purposes of your investigation and how you can proceed with your inquiries. With biases firmly in place, you won't have to pretend to complete objectivity, either' (p. 165).

One way to enhance this reflexive self-awareness is to utilise the services of a supportive but '*critical friend*' during a study. Their role is to provide a theoretical sounding board to encourage reflection upon, and exploration of, alternative explanations and interpretations of events in

182

the field and the analysis of the data as it is generated. An example is provided by Brewer and Sparkes (2011) in their ethnographic study of a community-based childhood bereavement organisation in the United Kingdom called the Rocky Centre. The purpose of their study was to explore the experiences of young people bereaved of a parent, and investigate the factors such as physical activity and sport that helped them to live with their grief. That Jo Brewer had been a former service user of the Rocky Centre was advantageous in terms of facilitating access. In other ways, however, it was problematic. This was particularly so with regard to the 'insider' being able to suspend common-sense understandings and make the 'familiar strange' in order to maintain analytical distance in settings where she or he is familiar with its norms, rules and ways of operating.

Accordingly, Andrew Sparkes, who had no connection with the Rocky Centre nor experienced childhood bereavement, played a key role throughout the study as a critical friend. Early on in the study, Andrew noticed that Jo was allowing her assumptions about the 'goodness' of the Rocky Centre to deflect her from asking critical questions about the ideologies informing its work and how these had developed and changed over time. At this stage, Andrew thought Jo was more of an 'advocate' for the Rocky Centre than an ethnographer seeking to understand it in all its complexity. This issue was the focus of a number of discussions with Jo and led her to undertake an archive analysis of the Rocky Centre to tease out the ideologies that informed its creation and early intervention strategies and how these had changed over time. Throughout the study, Andrew continued to ask Jo questions about how her own experiences of parental bereavement and the Rocky Centre might be influencing her reactions in the field and shaping her analysis of the data, in terms of how she came to know about the experiences of the participants. In this sense, Andrew acted as a continual 'bracketer' to Jo's thinking as the researcher in the field. This helped guard against the filters through which Jo viewed the world intruding on her capacity to engage with and listen to those involved in the Rocky Centre.

GENERALISATION

For Holloway (1997), generalisability (or external validity) in research is present when the findings of the study 'can be applied to other settings and cases or to a whole population, that is, when the findings are true beyond the focus of the work in hand' (p. 78). In quantitative research, generalisability is a standard aim and is normally achieved through statistical sampling procedures. Data in qualitative inquiry are often derived from one or more cases which are unlikely to have been selected on a random basis (see Chapters 1 and 3). As Silverman (2000) acknowledges, 'Moreover, even if you were able to construct a representative sample of cases, the sample size would be likely to be so large as to preclude the kind of intensive analysis usually preferred in qualitative research' (p. 102).

Qualitative researchers cannot make conventional *statistical* generalisations from cases to populations. Of course, given the logic, purposes and assumptions that inform their work, they do not wish to do so anyway. They utilise different forms of sampling and seek different forms of generalisations beyond the statistical kind. As Ruddin (2006) points out, 'It is exact that the case study is a detailed examination of a solitary exemplar, but it is false to utter that a case study cannot grant unswerving information about the broader class' (p. 797). Likewise, Collingridge and Gantt (2008: 2) comment, 'it is important to note that generalizability is not limited to probability sampling theory. There are different ways of understanding generalization'. There are, therefore, alternatives to statistical–probabilistic approaches to generalisation that are consistent with the non-random and purposeful sampling procedures used in qualitative research. For example, Yin (1989: 21) notes that case studies are generalisable to theoretical propositions and not to populations, or universes. For him, 'the case study, like the experiment, does not represent a "sample," and the investigator's goal is to expand and generalise theories (analytic generalisation) and not to enumerate frequencies (statistical generalisation)'.

Stake (1995: 85) makes a distinction between explicated (propositional) generalisations and what he calls *naturalistic* generalisations. These are 'conclusions arrived at though personal engagement in life's affairs or by vicarious experience so well constructed that the person feels as if it happened to themselves'. Here, the researcher is required to provide readers with rich, thick descriptions of the case under study so that *the readers themselves* can reflect upon it and make connections (that is, naturalistic generalisations) to their own situations.

Linked to naturalistic generalisation is Delmar's (2010) notion of *recognisability*. She acknowledges that the study of phenomena expressed through people's deliberations, experiences, decisions and actions is contingent on time, space, relations, power and context (including society and culture), but also that there will be typical traits and recognisable patterns available. For her, 'it is the experience from a similar situation that gives meaning. It is this recognisability that contributes to the 'generalisability' of qualitative studies' (p. 122). This takes place, Delmar argues, when the recipient of the new knowledge gives form to the recognisable and the typical by a practical transformation of the situation that they inhabit.

As Wolcott (1995: 172) notes about his own ethnographic work where the unit of study varied from one individual, to one village, and one institution, 'In each of those studies I make a few generalisations, implicate a few more, and leave readers the challenge of making further ones depending on their present concerns and prior experiences'. To assist the reader in making naturalistic generalisations from a case, Stake (1995) suggests the following.

> Researchers need to provide an opportunity for vicarious experience. Our accounts need to be personal, describing the things of our sensory experiences, not failing to attend to matters that personal curiosity dictates. A narrative account, a story, a chronological presentation, personalistic description, emphasis on time and place provide rich ingredients for vicarious experience.
>
> (Stake, 1995: 87)

Along similar lines, Lincoln and Guba (1985) and Guba and Lincoln (1994) developed their notions of transferability and fittingness as a parallel to the quantitative notion of external validity. Regarding the former they state that the qualitative researcher cannot specify the external validity of an inquiry but they can provide the thick description necessary to enable someone interested in making a transfer to reach a conclusion about whether such a transfer can be contemplated as a possibility.

> The degree of transferability is a direct function of the similarity between two [cases], what we shall call 'fittingness.' Fittingness is defined as the degree of congruence between sending and receiving contexts. If Context A and Context B are 'sufficiently' congruent then the working hypothesis from the sending originating context may be applicable to the receiving context.
>
> (Lincoln & Guba, 1985: 124)

More recently, in relation to creative analytical practices and the field of arts-based research in general (see Chapter 6), Barone and Eisner (2012) talk of *generativity*. This means the ways in which the work enables one to see or act upon phenomena even though it represents a case study of one. They emphasise that arts-based research is not primarily relevant for what can be measured and made statistical. For them, 'generalisations' take place all of the time without randomly selecting 'units' intended to represent some population and we generalise not only from an N = x but from a sample that is represented by N = 1.

> The arts typically project an image that reshapes our concep-
> tions of some aspect of the world or that sheds light on aspects
> of the world we had not seen before. Good arts based research
> generalises in such a fashion. It has 'legs' allowing us to go some-
> place. It does not simply reside in our own backyard forever but
> rather possesses the capacity to invite you into an experience that
> reminds you of people and places that bear familial resemblances
> to the settings, events, and characters within the work.
>
> (Barone & Eisner, 2012: 152)

The notions of naturalistic generalisation, transferability and generativity enable the consumers of qualitative research to examine the results of a study and make a judgment about whether to generalise this knowledge to other situations, including their own, without having to rely on statistical or probabilistic evidence. Developing such work, Chenail (2010) proposes that for qualitative researchers who choose to work within the generalisation framework, the alternative strategies available to them focus on either (a) generalising from a particular set of findings to a more general theory or (b) extrapolating knowledge in a case-to-case scenario.

In seeking to develop theory-focused generalisations, or what are sometimes called *analytical generalisations*, Chenail (2010) emphasises that the researcher strives to generalise a particular set of results to a broader theory. Researchers first examine relationships between the findings derived from the cases and a theory or theories. They then consider relationships between this theory, or theories, and other cases not directly studied in their primary research investigations. In contrast to the case-to-theory pattern evoked in analytical or theoretical generalisation, Chenail notes how case-to-case generalisation (or transfer) occurs whenever a person in one setting considers adopting something (for example, a programme or set of practices) from another. To facilitate the reader's ability to make this case-to-case generalisation, as noted earlier, the researcher needs to provide sufficient descriptive data to make such similarity judgments possible.

Reflecting on the methodological possibilities of analytical generalisations in qualitative research, Halkier (2011) discusses three different ways of generalising on the basis of the same qualitative data material. These are, *ideal typologising, category zooming* and *positioning*. Building ideal typologies seems to be one of the most frequently-used ways of producing analytical generalisations. The notion of ideal type comes from the work of Max Weber who defined this as a one-sidedly focused synthesis of diffuse and discrete empirical phenomena into a unified abstract analytical construct which will never be discovered in this specific form. In the process of building an ideal typology, Halkier warns that a considerable reduction of complexities takes place which runs the risk of excluding some themes and issues for others. He feels, therefore, it is a sensible option to make several different complementing claims from such data.

Another way of generalising on the basis of the same qualitative data material is through *category zooming*. This is different from ideal typologising 'in the sense that usually the inferences do not try to say something more comprehensive about the empirical patterns related centrally to the research question. Rather, this way of generalising goes into depth with the details and complexities of one single point in the study' (p. 792). A further way of making analytical generalisations on the basis of the same qualitative data material is through *positioning*. This form of generalisation, according to Halkier, underlines the non-stable and non-final character of inferences made on the basis of qualitative data material and should include and cover the communicative processes involved and their potential consequences for the contents of interpretation and analysis.

In reflecting on the different approaches to generalisability described above, Chenail (2010) comments on the different responsibilities ascribed to researchers and consumers of qualitative inquiry. In contrast to cases of probabilistic–statistical generalisability, where it is expected that the author is responsible for establishing the generalisability of the research, the proponents of theory-focused and case-to-case generalisability place the responsibility for judging the generalisability of the results on the reader/user. He notes that producers of research findings are also users of them and so this distinction is artificial. For him, 'researchers and con-sumers both share a responsibility when it comes to assessing the value of a particular set of qualitative research findings beyond the context and particulars of the original study' (p. 6). As Wolcott (1995) states when reflecting on his own work that usually involves case studies of one (per-son, village, or institution):

> What can we learn from studying only one of anything? Why, all we can! . . . If you want to know about an instance of something I have studied, my reports should be a rich resource, and that suggests a reasonable criterion by which to judge them. In each of these studies I make a few generalizations, implicate a few more, and leave to readers the challenge of making further ones depending on their present concerns and prior experiences.
>
> (Wolcott, 1995: 172)

In short, as Ruddin (2006) states in relation to qualitative research, 'You can generalise stupid!' It's just that the generalisations that can, and should be made from this form of inquiry are different from those aspired to in quantitative inquiry.

VALIDITY

Speaking from a quantitative perspective, Vaughn and Daniel (2012) note how the phrase 'the truthfulness of one's conclusions' encapsulates the general meaning of validity. They point out that in the context of measurement theory, 'there are several ways to view validity, but all are concerned with the confidence we can have regarding conclusions made from measurement instruments' (p. 33). A valid or truthful instrument measures what it is intended to measure. Internal and external validity, therefore, are appropriate concerns for quantitative researchers.

Traditionally, as Cho and Trent (2006: 320) suggest, validity in qualitative research involves determining 'the degree to which researchers' claims about knowledge correspond to the reality (or research participants' con-structions of reality)'. Likewise, Pitney and Parker (2009) state that the essence of internal validity is trust and accuracy. For them, 'the concept addresses whether research findings capture what really happened and what participants truly meant and believed about a situation' (p. 62). This said, validity in qualitative research is a messy concept with different claims being made for it in relation to phenomenological research (Vagle, 2011), hermeneutics and dialogic encounters (Freeman, 2011), and performance-related qualitative work (Cho & Trent, 2009). In short, qualitative researchers are divided about the application of validity to their work. Some of these divisions will become evident in what follows.

THE PARALLEL PERSPECTIVE

A common way of conceptualising validity in SEH has been to adopt a parallel perspective as described by Sparkes (1998, 2002a), or what Cho and Trent (2006) called a transactional notion of validity. Both have their roots in the work of Lincoln and Guba (1985: 301–328) and Guba and Lincoln (1989: 237–241) who suggest a *parallel* understanding of internal validity as *credibility* in which the focus moves to establishing the match between the constructed realities of respondents (or stakeholders) and those realities as represented by the evaluator and attributed to various stakeholders. To achieve the goal of credibility they suggest using a number of techniques that include the following:

- Prolonged engagement
- Persistent observation
- Triangulation (can include data–source triangulation, multiple-analyst triangulation, methodological triangulation and/or theoretical triangulation)
- Peer debriefing
- Negative case analysis
- Progressive subjectivity
- Member checks

In proposing the use of such techniques in relation to credibility, Lincoln and Guba situate themselves within what Cho and Trent (2006) call a 'transactional' notion of validity. The assumption is that qualitative research can be more credible as long as certain techniques, methods, and/or strategies are employed during the conduct of the study. These techniques are worthy of close attention by those conducting qualitative research. They have been well used within the field of SEH. For example, McDonough, Sabiston and Crocker (2008) in their phenomenologically-informed study of the psychosocial changes among breast cancer survivors involved in Dragon Boating, state that the principles of trustworthiness as outlined by Lincoln and Guba (1985) were used to evaluate their research. They then explain how they used selected techniques, such as having two investigators involved in every level of analysis, and providing substantial (thick) description, to achieve credibility, transferability, confirmability and dependability. Likewise, in their comparison of the developmental experiences of elite and sub-elite swimmers, Johnson, Tenebaum, Edmonds and Castillo (2011: 459–60) state that the methodological considerations that strengthened the trustworthiness of their study included the following, triangulating the data by interviewing the swimmer, one of his or her parents, and the athlete's coach; authenticating the interview transcripts via post-interview participant feedback; and having the data reviewed by multiple researchers.

THE PARALLEL PERSPECTIVE: A BRIEF CRITIQUE

In their critique of the parallel perspective on validity, Sparkes (1998, 2009b) and Sparkes and Smith (2009) noted the following problems: (1) There appears to be no explicit rationale to explain why certain techniques were chosen over others in various studies to establish trustworthiness; (2) Different meanings have been assigned to given techniques, such as member checking in different studies; (3) Some of the actual techniques proposed to achieve aspects of trustworthiness are not appropriate to the logic of qualitative research; (4) The parallel perspective is philosophically contradictory; (5) The parallel perspective supports a static form of criteriology; and (6) Lincoln and Guba changed their position towards the end of the 1980s and have continued to do so since (for example, see Lincoln, 2010). This raises questions about the non-reflective adherence to this earlier position adopted by many who conduct qualitative research in SEH.

Due to limitations of space we will only comment briefly on one of these problems, which revolves around member checking and which, according to Guba and Lincoln (1989), 'is the single most crucial technique for establishing credibility' (p. 239). Often called 'respondent validation' it involves the process of 'testing' working hypotheses, data, preliminary categories and interpretations with the participants involved in the study from whom the original constructions were collected. The researcher seeks to establish that the multiple realities that he or she presents are recognisable to the participants who provided them and that they agree it is an accurate interpretation of events. This process should be ongoing throughout the study but is crucial at the end of the study with regard to 'verifying' the findings.

190

Member checking as a method of verification is suspect for a number of reasons. It suggests that in the midst of multiple realities (that is, the researcher's and the participants'), that those being studied are the 'real knowers' and, therefore, the possessors of truth. There is, however, no reason to assume that participants have privileged status as commentators on their actions or motivations. As Day (2012: 64) argues, experience needs to be 'reflexively positioned within the broader social contexts in which they occur, so as to avoid the dilemma of experiential knowledge standing in for a claim to authority'. For her, we need to be careful not to replace the old 'tyranny of authoritarian expertise' that discounts people's lived experiences, with a new tyranny of 'experientialism' that makes first-person experiental utterances immune from challenge, interpretation and debate.

Participant feedback should not be granted an unquestioned authority in answering the question, 'who can know?' As Day (2012: 64) points out, an epistemological dilemma arises when we consider the possibility of competing knowledge claims based on experience. This is because 'we have no means to decide between contradictory claims to knowledge based on experience'. Therefore, participant feedback cannot be taken as a direct validation or refutation of the researcher's inferences. Rather, such processes, or so-called 'validation' techniques should be treated as yet another source of data and insight. Taking the findings back to the participants in the study are opportunities for reflexive elaboration and an enhanced understanding of how research findings are actually co-constructed in the creative process of the research and do not exist prior to it simply waiting to be discovered.

Finally, while member checking might be a useful strategy on some occasions it may not be so on all occasions. Goldblatt, Karnieli-Miller and Neumann (2011: 393) note that it can lead to ethical problems, especially in health care settings where, for example, 'A researcher who decides to share findings with participants may encounter dilemmas regarding the proper way to present the findings to allow participants to comment and criticise honestly, without threatening their personal world'. Goldblatt *et al.* warn that taking the findings and interpretations of events back to participants can lead to disappointment, hurt feelings and embarrassment for both participants and researchers. The participants may perceive researchers as being insensitive, and using their power to expose vulnerabilities. In these circumstances, researchers may feel that their ethical commitment to do no harm has been violated. Consequently, the original intent of gratitude and offering the participants the opportunity to learn and reflect about the self as well as have the chance to verify the researchers' interpretations are not achieved and become anxiety-inducing for all involved. Sharing qualitative findings or member checking is, therefore, a controversial and complex procedure that should be treated with caution and its use assessed carefully on a case by case basis in the light of the ethical dilemmas it poses for any given study (see Chapter 8). This is particularly so for research into sensitive and traumatic experiences.

This is not to say that procedures such as member checks are of no value. They can and do have value but only under certain conditions and in certain situations depending upon the specific purposes of the inquiry. The choice about procedures in any instance depends on what seems to be important at the time. It remains, however, that methods or techniques alone will *not* sort out the trustworthy from the untrustworthy and, as we emphasise later, applying a set of universal evaluative criteria to all qualitative projects is not possible.

THE DIVERSIFICATION PERSPECTIVE

Various scholars working within what Sparkes (1998, 2002a) calls a *diversification perspective* and Cho and Trent (2006) call a *transformational* approach have opted to radically reconceptualise or reframe the notion of validity for the purposes of judging different forms of inquiry. In particular, for those qualitative researchers whose work is informed by a critical agenda that is openly ideological, the issue of validity takes on various meanings that revolve around the resultant actions prompted by the research endeavour. Thus there is talk of *catalytic validity* which refers to the degree to which the research process energised participants and altered their consciousness so that they know reality better in order to transform it.

Guba and Lincoln's (2005: 207) notion of *catalytic* and *tactical authenticities* also refers to the ability of a given inquiry to prompt, 'first, action on the part of the participants and, second, the involvement of the researcher/evaluator in training participants in specific forms of social and political action if participants desire the training'. Validity in critical research, therefore, might involve some evaluation of how effective the research process, and the research product in the form of text, has been in actually empowering the participants and enabling them to cre-

192

ate change. That is, has the research made a difference? Has it moved people to action? Has it challenged and changed power differentials and structures?

Richardson (2000) also offered a transgressive take on validity by reconceptualising it in terms of the *crystalline*. That is, validity, in a metaphoric sense, has the properties of a crystal rather than the fixed points assumed within methods triangulation:

> The central imaginary is the crystal which combines symmetry and substance with an infinite variety of shapes, substances, transmutations, multidimensionalities, and angles of approach ... Crystals are prisms that reflect externalities *and* refract within themselves, creating different colors, patterns, and arrays, casting off in different directions. What we see depends upon our angle of repose. Not triangulation, crystallization.
>
> (Richardson, 2000: 934)

Crystallisation suggests that we might draw on multiple ways of judging qualitative forms of inquiry using different forms of validity that might vary over time, depending upon the angle of repose, for the same piece of research. Therefore, we need to think not of a singular validity but of validities as diverse conceptualisations that are associated with different qualitative research traditions.

The diversification perspective is useful as it provides qualitative researchers with a new vocabulary regarding validity. In seeking to tell a different story about the process and product of research, however, it remains parasitic on the old terminology. Thus, the term 'validity' is retained while modifiers, such as 'catalytic', are added. For Scheurich (1997) this approach is problematic. He argues that by holding on to the term validity, even those who seek a radical reconstruction of its meanings are fighting a lost cause due to the cultural baggage this term carries with it. Validity acts as a boundary marker or serves a policing function across both conventional approaches and more radical alternatives, so that an unsettling and disturbing sameness prevails across paradigms that reproduces the 'same Western preconceptual presumption (or map) – something is either warranted (trustworthy) or not warranted (untrustworthy)' (pp. 87–88).

More recently, problems associated with the diversification perspective in terms of its impact on the long-term development of qualitative research have beejn voiced. For example, Koro-Ljungberg (2010) elaborates on how the label of validity and its identifiers function, are understood, and are used. As part of this elaboration a form of validation in the making is described that is based on epistemological and methodological exclusionism. This is contrasted to a more pluralistic approach to *validation*, rather than validity, that acknowledges the diverse ways of making, conducting, and legitimising research. From this perspective validity and validation are possibilities and processes that enable scholars to establish various knowledge claims rather than to execute an objective evaluation of truth. For Koro-Ljungberg, all validity and validation definitions are limited and partial so that all domimant and narrow conceptions of each need to be questioned and alternative perspectives welcomed.

THE LETTING GO PERSPECTIVE

Reacting to the parallel and diversification perspectives on validity as described above, some researchers, as part of what Sparkes (1998, 2002a) calls a *letting go* perspective, have chosen to abandon the notion of validity completely. Indeed, Wolcott (1994) talks of the 'absurdity of validity':

> What I seek is something else, a quality that points more to identifying critical elements and wringing plausible interpretations from them, something one can pursue without becoming obsessed with finding the right or ultimate answer, the correct version, the Truth . . . And I do not accept validity as a valid criterion for guiding or judging my work. I think we have labored far too long under the burden of this concept (are there others as well?) that might have been better left where it began, a not-quite-so-singular-or-precise criterion as I once believed it to be for matters related essentially to tests and measurement. I suggest we look elsewhere in our continuing search for and dialogue about criteria appropriate to qualitative researchers' approaches and purposes.
>
> (Wolcott, 1994: 366–369)

Likewise, reflecting on the purposes of autoethnography, Allen-Collinson (2012) states, 'For those seeking to adhere to the traditional triad of evaluation criteria appropriate to the scientific methods – validity, reliability and generalisability – autoethnographic research would not provide a suitable methodology, and indeed has no concern with fulfilling these criteria' (p. 206). For her and other qualitative researchers, particularly those involved in creative analytical practices, such as those decribed in Chapter 6, this 'looking elsewhere' for appropriate criteria has led them to examine how judgments are passed in the arts and the developing field of arts-based research (Barone & Eisner, 2012; Knowles & Cole, 2008; Sparkes, 2002a, 2009b).

Judgments about social research, Smith and Hodkinson (2009: 35) believe, are much more akin to judgments about the quality of works of 'music, painting, literature, and so on, which depend on time- and place-contingent lists of characteristics, than they are to the time- and place-independent "connect to reality" judgments in the physical sciences'. Supporting this view, Barone and Eisner (2012) argue that as opposed to standards that employ quantitative metrics to enumerate or establish quantity, criteria demand judgments regarding significance or value. They point out that art critics do not seek a universal standard for making judgements about the quality of a work. Rather, what they seek are achievements related to whatever the criteria that are appropriate for that particular work to be assessed:

> The particular criteria that are applicable to a work depend, at least in some measure, on the particular character of the work. Appraising the quality of a skater doing figure eights requires criteria that are quite different than those applied to the same skater doing improvisational dance on ice.
>
> (Barone & Eisner, 2012: 147)

Criteria used for judging a grounded-theory study as opposed to a phenomenological study, or an ethnodrama/theatre, are likely to be different. Such a *relativist* view stands in opposition to the criteriological approach contained within the parallel perspective and is wary of any attempt to determine specific universal judgement criteria in advance of any particular piece of inquiry. For the latter, in passing judgment, it is necessary to appeal to time- and place-contingent lists of characteristics to sort out the good from the not-so-good in qualitative research.

Sparkes (2002a, 2009b) and Sparkes and Smith (2009) emphasise that this form of relativism does not mean that 'anything goes' when it comes to making assessments about the quality of an inquiry. Nor does it mean that all knowledge claims are equal to other knowledge claims. Smith and

Deemer (2000) point out that relativists can and do make judgements and will continue to do so for the foreseeable future. For them, just because these judgements cannot be grounded extralinguistically does not mean that we are exempt from engaging in as

> open and unconstrained dialogue as possible in order to attempt to justify our assessments . . . All relativism brings to the table with regard to the issue of criteria is that to be a finite human being who must live with and make judgements with other finite human beings can be, with some frequency, very tough work indeed.
>
> (p. 885)

From a relativistic point of view, when passing judgement on a piece of research, criteria are not taken to mean an absolute or preordained standard against which to make judgment. This position is laden with foundational implications which then become a touchstone that can be employed to distinguish the good from the bad, the correct from the incorrect. Rather, relativists adhere to the view proposed by Smith (1993) that criteria are *characterising traits* that have, at best, mild implications as a prescription for inquirer behaviour and do not necessarily refer to something that is held to be foundational. From this perspective, researchers might discuss the characterising traits of a particular qualitative approach to inquiry and simply note that these criteria are the way researchers seem to be conducting their particular kind of inquiries at the moment. The difference here from the criteriological and foundational view is that those holding a relativistic position are willing to describe what one *might* do, but are not prepared to mandate what one *must* do across all contexts and on all occasions prior to any piece of research being conducted.

For Smith (1993), and Smith and Deemer (2000), once criteria come to be seen as characterising traits or values that influence our judgments, then any particular traits or values will always be subject to constant reinterpretation as times and conditions change. They have a list-like quality. Saying this, we do not wish to imply that the more criteria achieved on any given list, the better the quality of the study. Matching ten criteria from a list does not necessarily make the study twice as good as a study that 'only' matches five criteria.

> The use of the term *list* should not be taken to mean that we are referring to something like an enclosed and precisely specified or specifiable shopping or laundry list. Put differently, to talk of a list

196

in this sense is not at all to talk about, for example, an accumulation of 20 items, scaled 1–5, where everyone's presentation proposal is then numerically scored with a cut off point for acceptance. Obviously, to think of a list in these terms is to miss the entire point.

(Smith & Deemer, 2000: 888)

In contrast, Smith and Deemer (2000), and Smith and Hodkinson (2005) see any list of characteristics as always open-ended, and ever subject to constant reinterpretation so that items can be added to the list or taken away. They emphasise that the items on the list cannot be derived from a distillation of some abstract epistemology but rather derive from the standpoint we adopt on any given issue. Therefore, the criteria used to judge a piece of research can change depending upon the context and the purposes. This is because a characteristic of research we thought important at one time and in one place may take on diminished importance at another time and place. As Kerry-Moran (2008) states in relation to evaluating arts-related research, 'perspectives, climates, cultures, and goals change. Any attempt to evaluate the quality of the arts in research must balance shared perspectives of art-related inquiry with the unique attributes and purposes of particular approaches, projects, or products' (p. 498).

Given the situation as described, and in keeping with the 'letting go' perspective, a number of scholars in recent years have suggested various lists of criteria for judging qualitative work in general, and certain traditions in particular. The following are but a few examples. Tracy (2010: 840) offers the following eight 'big-tent' criteria for judging excellence in qualitative research and provides various means, practices and methods through which these might be achieved:

- *Worthy topic*: The topic of the research is relevant, timely, significant, interesting, or evocative.
- *Rich rigor*: The study uses sufficient, abundant, appropriate, and complex theoretical constructs, data and time in the field, sample(s), context(s), and data collection and analysis processes.
- *Sincerity*: The study is characterised by self-reflexivity about subjective values, biases and inclinations of the researcher(s); and transparency about methods and challenges.
- *Credibility*: The research is marked by thick description, concrete detail, explication of tacit (nontextual) knowledge, and showing rather than telling; triangulation or crystallisation; multivocality; and member reflections.

- *Resonance*: The research influences, affects, or moves particular readers or a variety of readers through aesthetic, evocative representations; naturalistic generalisations; and transferable findings.
- *Significant contribution*: The research provides a significant contribution conceptually/theoretically, practically, morally, methodologically and heuristically.
- *Ethical*: The research considers procedural ethics (such as human subjects); situational and culturally specific ethics; relational ethics; and exiting ethics (leaving the scene and sharing the research).
- *Meaningful coherence*: The study achieves what it purports to be about; uses methods and procedures that fit its stated goals; and meaningfully interconnects literature, research questions/foci, findings and interpretations with each other.

With regard to autoethnography, Holman Jones (2005: 773) offers the following list of criteria:

- *Participation as reciprocity*: How well does the work construct participation of authors/readers and performer/audiences as a reciprocal relationship marked by mutual responsibility and obligation?
- *Partiality, reflexivity and citationality as strategies for dialogue (and not 'mastery')*: How well does the work present a partial and self-referential tale that connects with other stories, ideas, discourses and contexts (for example, personal, theoretical, ideological, cultural) as a means of creating a dialogue among authors, readers, and subjects written/read?
- *Dialogue as a space of debate and negotiation*: How well does the work create a space for and engage in meaningful dialogue among different bodies, hearts and minds?
- *Personal narrative and storytelling as an obligation to critique*: How do narrative and story enact an ethical obligation to critique subject positions, acts, and received notions of expertise and justice within and outside of the work?
- *Evocation and emotion as incitements to action.* How well does the work create a plausible and visceral lifeworld and charged emotional atmosphere as an incitement to act within and outside the context of the work?
- *Engaged embodiment as a condition for change.* How does the work place/embody/interrogate/intervene in experience in ways that make political action and change possible in and outside the work?

198

In relation to judging arts-based research Barone and Eisner (2012: 148–154) suggest the following six criteria:

- *Incisiveness*: Research that gets to the heart of a social issue. It goes to its core. It does not get swamped with details that have no inherent significance and do little to increase the cogency of the research itself. Incisiveness means that the work of research is penetrating; it is sharp in the manner in which it cuts to the core of an issue.

- *Concision*: Pertains to the degree to which the arts based research occupies the minimal amount of space or includes the least amount of verbiage necessary for it to serve its primary, heuristic purpose of enabling members of the audience to see social phenomena from a fresh perspective.

- *Coherence*: The creation of a work of arts based research whose features hang together as a strong form. Gestalt psychologists often refer to the law of *pragnanz*, a law that pertains to the way components in a complex form hang together. Does the short story hang together so that the reader has a sense of completion in reading the story? Does the painting 'work'? Does it represent a 'good gestalt'?

- *Generativity*: The ways in which the work enables one to see or act upon phenomena even though it represents a kind of case study with an N of only 1.

- *Social significance*: Significance pertains to the character, meaning and import of the central ideas of the work. What makes a work significant is its thematic importance, its focus on the issues that make a sizeable difference in the lives of people within society. What one is looking for is something that matters, ideas that count, important questions to be raised.

- *Evocation and illumination*: It is through evocation and illumination that one begins to *feel* the meanings that the work is to help its readers grasp . . . Paintings are read, music is read, and dance is read. Evocation is therefore an epistemological means for the acquisition of meaning . . . It may signify an aesthetic experience . . . 'Illumination' as applied to arts based research pertains to the ways in which the work illuminates a terrain, a process, and individual. It sheds light often by defamiliarising an object or a process so that it can be seen in a way that is entirely different than a way in which customary modes of perception operate.

In proposing their lists, the scholars named above are quick to point out that they do not wish to imply that these are the *only* criteria that can be used for passing judgement. Rather, the criteria are suggestions that can be added to or subtracted from depending on purpose. While they recognise that there is utility in commonality, they understand that there is also liability in that one can get locked into criteria in ways that constrain innovation and dampen the imagination. To guard against this static form of criteriology it would seem sensible not to determine in an exclusionary manner a list of criteria prior to engaging with a piece of inquiry but rather the list should be developed in the engagement itself. As Holman Jones (2005: 773) notes, 'I have developed a list of actions and accomplishments that I look for in the work of others. They are changing. They are generated in the doing of this writing rather than outside or prior to it'. Again, it is important to emphasise that the importance we assign to items on our list may easily change over time:

> As we approach judgment in any given case, we have in mind a list of characteristics that we use to judge the quality of that production. This is not a well defined and precisely specified list; to the contrary, this list of characteristics is always open-ended, in part unarticulated, and always subject to constant interpretation and reinterpretation.
>
> (Smith & Hodkinson, 2005: 922)

Criteria that might have been thought of as important at one time in another place may take on diminished importance at another time and place. The list gets challenged and changed not by abstracted discussions but by the application and engagement with actual inquiries, and the practical wisdom gained through experience (that is, *phronesis*). As Smith and Deemer (2000: 889) point out, novel forms of inquiry can offer serious challenges and immediately opens up the 'possibility that one must reformulate one's list and possibly replace the exemplars one calls upon in the never-ending process of making judgements'. Even though she apparently defines universal criteria for judging qualitative research, Tracy (2010: 849) acknowledges that understanding qualitative goodness is best appreciated by engaging with the complexities of the research process itself. For her, 'while rules and guidelines are helpful, if it were really as straightforward as 'eight simple criteria', there would be no magic, no surprises, and therefore no genius'.

200

Barone and Eisner (2012) emphasise that each of the criteria they have included in their list for judging arts-based research function as *cues for perception*. They offer these criteria as starting points for thinking about the appraisal of works of arts-based research. While their criteria may act as a common point of reflection, Barone and Eisner do not want these to be seen as a fixed recipe that all must follow as this will lead to rigid standardisation at the cost of innovation.

> So, finally, we invite you, the readers, to use your own judgement in applying these criteria to the examples of the works of arts-based research included in this book and to those many that are not included. But we also urge you to use your imagination in ascertaining other criteria that may emerge from your encounters with arts-based work in the future.
>
> (Barone & Eisner, 2012: 154–155)

Given that standards can and do change within fields of inquiry, any notion of criteria needs to be seen as process-orientated and emergent in nature as opposed to fixed and permanent. As new forms of understanding and representing the world of SEH develop so new ways of passing judgment will be required. Therefore, as Koro-Ljungberg (2008) argues, 'The more we know about particularities and other conceptualisations of validity and validation, the more informed we will be when making decisions regarding validity and validation in our projects, as well as the research studies we read' (p. 988). Likewise, qualitative researchers have a duty to engage in the continuing task of creating new criteria for choosing criteria in relation to their work.

WORKING WITH LISTS

For certain purposes and types of inquiry, the trustworthiness criteria proposed by Lincoln and Guba (1985) may be appropriate and the researcher should provide a rationale for their use, and the techniques chosen over others in the list available to achieve these criteria. For other researchers with different purposes in mind the same criteria might be deemed inappropriate. In this instance, researchers might choose all or some of the criteria given in the list by Tracy (2010) as relevant to their work. Alternatively, researchers might select some criteria from each list provided earlier if they feel these are relevant to their work. That is, criteria from lists can be mixed and matched as required as long as the choices made are discussed in detail as part of a coherent rationale for the study. This point is emphasised by Cho and Trent (2006) in their attempt to develop an inclusive discourse on validity in qualitative research that is open to the bricolage of a variety of approaches.

> Our distinction is that it is not an either/or choice. One need not choose between practical and emancipatory purposes any more than one must select transactional validity criteria over trans-formational validity aims. Transformational approaches seeking ameliorative change can and should be combined, when deemed relevant by the researcher(s) and/or participants, with more traditional trustworthiness-like criteria.
>
> (Cho & Trent, 2006: 333)

In this regard, it is interesting to note how some scholars within the SEH who have utilised novel forms of representation have adopted the strategy of selecting from various lists the criteria they feel are relevant to their work and then making these explicit to the readers. For example, Carless and Sparkes (2008) provide a list of criteria to assist the reader judge their use of three short stories to explore the experiences of a small group of men with severe mental illness as they engage in exercise. Sparkes and Douglas (2007) also provide a list of criteria to assist the reader judge their poetic representations of the experiences of an elite woman golfer, called Leanne, and her decision to retire early from the sport. These include the following: Do the poetic representations succeed aesthetically? Do they invite a range of interpretive responses? Do they create evocative and open-ended connections to the data? Are they effective in relation to its intended purposes and audiences? Do they evoke the emotional dimensions of Leanne's experiences? Do they generate new questions about motivational issues? Have they raised the level of awareness of Leanne and the other research participants, and have they also raised the awareness of the individuals who surround them and shape their experiences within their sports organisations. Did Leanne have a chance to contribute and share her views as part of the process? Did she find the representation of her to be fair and respectful?

More recently, in relation to the transformation of the stories of Australian swimmers about their body practices into an ethnodrama, McMahon, Penny and Dinan-Thompson (2012) name the following criteria as useful for judging their work: verisimilitude, evocation and enlightenment. With regard to evocation they note their intention to provide the reader

> with a bona fide sense of what it was like to be involved at both an elite and amateur level of Australian sport, and reveal intimate details privy only to those few individuals immersed in the Australian swimming culture to provoke an emotional response in the reader; to penetrate readers' 'heads and hearts'.
>
> (McMahon et al., 2012: 185)

As both Carless and Sparkes (2008), and Sparkes and Douglas (2007) emphasise, the lists of criteria they provide are intended to act as starting points for judging their poetic representations and short stories as a mode of analysis and communication rather than as standardised templates for use on all occasions. Other scholars, and indeed themselves, with different purposes on different occasions might choose to have different criteria in their list. This selection and justification of criteria needs to be seen as part of the informed, principled and strategic decision-making involved in any form of qualitative research endeavour.

The principled decision-making process we have advocated requires that those working in different traditions along with the consumers of research are able and willing to engage with alternative notions of 'goodness' and the various criteria available for assessing this notion in practice. As Sparkes (2002a, 2009b) argues, this is necessary if the differences between alternative forms of inquiry, in terms of their process and products, are to be acknowledged so that each can be judged in a fair and respectful manner using criteria that are consistent with their own internal meaning structures and purposes. Without this willingness, he warns, the criteriological tendency is to impose preordained criteria on all forms of inquiry regardless of purpose. The end result of this process, Sparkes suggests, is to build in failure from the start for non-traditional forms of inquiry so that their legitimacy and the contribution they can make to our ways of knowing and understanding are systematically denied.

Acknowledging and respecting difference, and stepping outside one's zone of comfort and expertise to engage with alternative judgment criteria, is no easy task. It requires a complex conceptual shift in the way one approaches issues of difference in judging research in general and different forms of representation in particular. Furthermore, the realisation of difference creates an ethical imperative in which the task, according to

Bernstein (1991: 66), is to assume the responsibility to listen carefully and attempt to grasp what is being expressed and said in alien traditions. For him, such responsibility 'should not be confused with an indifferent superficial tolerance where no effort is made to understand and engage with the incommensurable otherness of the "Other"'.

Assuming the responsibility to listen carefully, and attempting to grasp what is being expressed in different traditions so that judgment might be passed in an ethical and fair manner, according to Sparkes (2009b) and Sparkes and Smith (2009) calls for the qualities of *connoisseurship*. For Eisner (1991: 63) this involves the ability to make fine-grained discriminations among complex and subtle qualities: 'Connoisseurship is the art of appreciation. It can be displayed in any realm in which the character, import, or value of objects, situations, and performances is distributed and variable'. He emphasised that the term *appreciation* should not be conflated with 'a liking for'. That is, there is no necessary relationship between appreciating something and liking it. Eisner states that, 'Nothing in connoisseurship as a form of appreciation requires that our judgements be positive. What is required (or desired) is that our experience be subtle, complex, and informed' (p. 69).

Connoisseurship, therefore, is about risking one's prejudices when encountering something new or unfamiliar. As Smith and Deemer (2000: 889) comment, 'Just as in the process of judgement one asks questions of a text or person, the person or text must be allowed to ask questions in return'. They argue that approaching a novel piece of work requires that one be willing to allow the text to challenge one's prejudices and possibly change the criteria one is using to judge the piece, thereby changing one's idea of what is and is not good inquiry. Smith and Deemer are quick to point out that to be open does not mean to accept automatically, and that one may still offer reasons for not accepting something new. The outcome of any judgment is uncertain. Furthermore, they stress there is no *method* for engaging in the risking of one's prejudices and, if anything, 'to risk one's prejudices is a matter of disposition – or, better said, moral obligation – that requires one to accept that if one wishes to persuade others, one must be equally open to be persuaded' (p. 889).

SUMMARY

In this chapter we have examined what the concepts of reliability, objectivity, generalisability and validity might mean in qualitative research.

judging the quality of qualitative research

We have shown that the meanings attached to each of these terms is varied and that qualitative researchers of different persuasions have addressed them in different ways. This being particularly so with regard to the issue of validity and how it has been dealt within a parallel, a diversification, and a letting go perspective. As part of this exploration we promoted the idea of criteria as characterising traits that might best be developed in a list-like fashion as a practical mode of engagement according to the purposes of any given study. As Denzin (2010) reminds us:

> You can only critique a work from within its paradigm. It makes no sense to apply foundational–positivistic criteria to a poem, or to performance ethnography. In turn performance criteria should not be applied to a piece of statistical analysis. The two projects rest on different politics of representation. To repeat: differences in interpretive criteria must be honored.
>
> (Denzin, 2010: 41)

Given the variety of criteria now available to judge qualitative research in SEH, we suggested that consumers, if they are to make fair and ethical judgments on different kinds of qualitative research, need to develop the qualities of connoisseurship. In this sense, criteria are useful pedagogical tools to help us learn, practice and engage with the various traditions within qualitative research and form a basis for communication across traditions and across paradigms. As Tracy (2010: 837) reminds us, 'Values for quality, like all social knowledge, are ever changing and situated within local contexts and current conversations. As such, it is important to regularly dialogue about what makes good qualitative research'. In this chapter, therefore, we have provided the reader with the material to challenge both their own prejudices and the prejudices of others when it comes to judging the goodness of qualitative research. We hope that in so doing they will be encouraged to engage in dialogue across difference as part of the process of becoming a reflexive qualitative researcher in SEH.

CHAPTER 8

ETHICAL ISSUES IN QUALITATIVE RESEARCH

As indicated in Chapter 3, as part of a pre-study task, gaining ethical clearance from a Research Ethics Committee (REC) or an Institutional Review Board (IRB) is a necessary first step in the qualitative research journey. It is not, however, the only step. It is not sufficient to assume that simply because ethical approval has been sought and granted by a committee, or that research is being conducted within the auspices of an organisation with a clear code of ethics, that a research project will have satisfied all the requirements of ethical research. Ethics is not a static event but a continual process. A number of ethical positions can be adopted and each have important implications for how qualitative researchers go about their work from start to finish. Some of these and how they deal with key issues will be considered in this chapter.

TRADITIONAL ETHICAL POSITIONS

We begin with two traditional positions that involve a form of *procedural ethics,* both of which inform the work of RECs and IRBs. The first position is known as *utilitarian* or *utilitarian consequentialism.* This is a position driven by a belief in universal ethical principles and replaces metaphysical distinctions with the calculation of empirical quantities. In terms of making judgments of 'rightness' or 'goodness' this position emphasises the consequences or results of an action (for example, increased knowledge or happiness) rather than its intent. The end purpose – the morally right course of action in any situation – is the one that produces the greatest good for the greatest number. Thus, in utilitarianism the locus of right and wrong is placed solely on the consequences of choosing one action over other actions. For Mauthner, Birch, Miller and Jessop (2012), this position is informed by a universalistic cost–benefit result pragmatism that, *in extremis*, can lead to a situation where the ends come to justify the means. Furthermore, notes Christians (2005), with utilitarian ethics, autonomous reason is the arbiter of moral disputes.

206

Another traditional position on ethics is termed *principlism* (Blee and Currier, 2011), or a *duty ethics of principles* (Mauthner *et al.* 2012). Like utilitarianism it is driven by universal principles, such as honesty, justice and respect, that can be applied in all circumstances and should never be broken. As Kvale and Brinkmann (2009) point out, however, principlism differs from utilitarianism in that actions are judged by their *intent* rather than their consequences. This notion of intent and the position of principlism strongly influences the current regulation of human subjects research by RECs and IRBs who seek to ensure procedures that adequately deal with autonomy, justice, informed consent, confidentiality, right to privacy, deception and protecting human subjects from harm.

Both utilitarianism and principlism are what Lahman, Geist, Rodriguez, Graglia and DeRoche (2011) define as *minimalist* or mandatory codes which are informed by a form of procedural ethics that focuses on participants' rights and the outcomes of the research. While such minimalist ethical codes cover foundational concerns, Lahman and her colleagues argue that research ethics should move beyond these codes 'due both to the irrepressible nature of all human research and to the in-depth, long-term relationships that may develop between participants and researchers in some forms of human research' (p. 1399). This 'movement beyond' has been stimulated by a number of challenges to minimalist and universalistic codes of ethics that have been mounted by scholars associated with all the qualitative traditions mentioned in Chapter 2 and, in particular, by those engaged in openly ideological research. Drawing on the work of Cannella and Lincoln (2011), Denzin, 1997, 2010), and Mauthner *et al.* (2012) these challenges to the minimalist and universalistic codes of ethics may be summarised as follows:

- They are monological, defining people as bounded, autonomous self-contained subjects rather than as dialogical and relational.
- They remain modernist, male-orientated, and imperialist.
- They neglect oppression, privilege, and care-based practices, ignoring the situatedness of power relations associated with gender, age, class, sexual orientation, disability, race, ethnicity, and nationality.
- They are an illusion in presuming a morally neutral researcher or value-free observer that is not feasible.
- Ethical decisions are largely assumed to be independent of culture, the particular, the biographical, of time, and of place.

- They rest on a cognitive model that privileges rational solutions to ethical dilemmas (the rationalist fallacy), and presume that humanity is a single subject (the distributive fallacy).
- No universally shared ethical model has been found to work.

At a more basic level concerns have been expressed about how RECs and IRBs operate when driven by utilitarianism and principlism. Drawing on the work of Franklin *et al.* (2012), Green and Thorogood (2009), Hammersley (2009), and O'Reilly (2012) these concerns can be summarised as follows:

- They tend to use a regulatory model of research ethics based on the positivist tradition of biomedical research, which assumes the existence of objective, universal truths and an 'essentialised' subject.
- They will have expertise in selected areas and methodologies (usually quantitative) and but may have little experience in judging the appropriateness of qualitative designs.
- They may lack the ability to understand the nature of ethics as an emergent process in the field.
- While their value in formally protecting participants is recognised, the institutional machinery that has now evolved to protect participants has turned into a bureaucratic nightmare designed ultimately to protect only the institutions themselves.
- They reduce ethical principles to a requirement that researchers comply with bureaucratic procedures which fails to engage researchers in a meaningful discussion about moral choices.
- They are *incapable* of making sound – and, even less, *superior* – ethical decisions about particular research projects.
- Their heavy regulation discourages ground-breaking, flexible, difficult, and sensitive work and stunts the development of innovative, exciting and valuable research because the ethical issues seem too difficult to resolve.
- Many of the most important and complex issues involved in the doing of field work lie beyond their remit.

Against this backdrop, Wolcott (2002) recommends the following tactic:

> The best advice I can offer to researchers confronting formal review procedures – and these days this includes virtually all researchers – is to treat the bureaucratic process with about as

ethical issues in qualitative research

much reverence as you would renewing your driver's license. Do what you have to do, tell them what you need to tell them (that is, what they need to hear), and get on with it. Ethics are not housed in such procedures.

(Wolcott, 2002: 148)

ALTERNATIVE ETHICAL POSITIONS

A number of alternative ethical positions to the minimalist codes and universalism of utilitarianism and principlism have emerged. Collectively, Lahman *et al.* (2011) describe these alternatives as *aspirational* ethics which are 'the highest stance the researcher tries to attain in ethics above and beyond minimum requirements. Researchers' aspirational ethical stances may differ depending on culture, values and morals, and are judged and processed internally with no mandated checks' (p. 1400). They give the following examples of such aspirational stances: relational ethics, feminist ethics, virtue ethics, narrative ethics, covenantal ethics, ethics in practice, caring ethics, and situational ethics. Some of these will now be considered.

Virtue ethics conceives ethical behaviour not so much as the application of abstract rules or universal principles but instead as contextual or situational. The emphasis is on *phronesis*, that is, cultivated practical wisdom (Kvale & Brinkmann, 2009). It stresses the researcher's moral values and skills in reflexively negotiating ethical dilemmas. As Mauthner *et al.* (2012) point out, the ethical intuitions, feelings and reflexive skills of researchers are emphasised, including their sensibilities in undertaking dialogue and negotiation with the various parties involved in the research. Likewise, Blee and Currier (2011) note that in virtue ethics the focus is on the agent, rather than the act, of research. Ethical research 'is done by ethical persons or researchers with integrity who have such characteristics as courage, honesty, resoluteness, and humility' (p. 403). In this position changing individuals' behaviours with others to promote more ethical action and to forestall ethical mishaps is emphasised.

Feminist scholars have proposed another ethical position that emphasises care and responsibility rather than just outcomes. This position focuses on particular feminist-informed social values that revolve around personal experience, context and nurturing relationships. According to Blee and Currier (2011), rather than searching for neutral principles to which everyone can appeal, *feminist ethics* is located in moral understandings within a larger framework of social relationships. They note that morality 'is part of ongoing social life, not solely a function of philosophical thought' (p. 403). Speaking of feminist ethics, Steiner (2009) notes the following features:

> Feminist approaches to ethics challenge women's subordination, prescribe morally justifiable ways of resisting oppressive practices, and envision morally desirable alternatives that promote emancipation . . . Fully feminist ethics, far more than their feminine and material counterparts, are distinctly political . . . A feminist approach to ethics asks questions about power even before it asks questions about good and evil, care and justice, or material and paternal thinking. With feminism's persuasive critique of the disembodied ethical subject generating a healthy respect for difference, a muliculturalist feminism may yet construct a non-sexist theory that represents difference of all sorts.
>
> (Steiner, 2009: 377)

Various approaches exist within feminist ethics. For example, feminists like Cannella and Lincoln (2011) support a *critical research ethics* that values and recognises the need to expose the diversity of realities and engage with the webs of interaction that create problems in ways that lead to power or privilege for certain groups. It seeks also to reposition decisions and problems toward social justice and join 'in solidarity with the traditionally oppressed to create new ways of functioning' (p. 83). Linked to this, Christians (2005) and Denzin (1997) propose a *feminist, communitarian* model of ethics.

> This is a normative model that serves as an antidote to individualist utilitarianism. It presumes that the community is ontologically and axiologically prior to persons. Human identity is constituted through the social realm. We are born into a sociocultural universe where values, moral commitments, and existential meanings are negotiated dialogically. Fulfilment is never achieved in isolation, but only though human bonding at the epicentre of social formation . . . What is worth preserving as good cannot be self-determined in isolation, but can be ascertained only within specific social situations where human identity is nurtured . . . Morally appropriate action intends community. Common moral values are intrinsic to a community's ongoing existence and identity.
>
> (Christians, 2005: 150–151)

In this approach, research is intended to be collaborative in its design and participatory in its execution. The participants are involved in determining what constitutes an ethical stance in their particular situation and how and when ethical procedures might be enacted and with whom. Importantly, as Christians (2005) points out, 'the substantive conceptions of the good that drive the problems reflect the conceptions of the community rather than the expertise of researchers or funding agencies' (p. 151).

An associated feminist approach described by Edwards and Mauthner (2012) is that of a *feminist ethics of care*. For them, ethics is about how to deal with difference, disagreement, conflict and ambivalence rather than attempting to eliminate it. They offer the following set of questions as a form of contingent guidelines for ethical practice informed by a feminist ethics of care:

- Who are the people (for example, researcher, participants, funders and gate-keepers) involved in and affected by the ethical dilemmas raised in the research?
- What is the context for the dilemma in terms of the specific topic of the research and the issues it raises personally and socially for those involved?
- What are the specific social and personal locations of the people involved in relation to each other?
- What are the needs of those involved and how are they inter-related?
- What am I identifying with, who am I posing as other, and why?
- What is the balance of personal and social power between those involved?
- How will those involved understand our actions and these in balance with our judgment about our own practice?
- How can we best communicate the ethical dilemmas to those involved, give them room to raise their views, and negotiate with and between them?
- How will our actions affect relationships between the people involved? (Edwards and Mauthner, 2012: 28–29)

Another aspirational ethical position advocated by Lahman *et al.* (2011) is that of *culturally responsive relational reflexive ethics* (CRRRE). They suggest a stance which acknowledges that researchers will not be able to fully understand the perspective of the varied cultures with whom they interact and, therefore, recognises the need to be 'flexible and open to studying ethical issues from the perspective of the participants to the extent possible' (p. 1401). CRRRE calls for researchers to integrate in practice three interrelated 'R's of ethics:

Culturally responsive ethics: Researchers must be aware of the cultures in which they are personally embedded and then attempt to understand and affirm others' cultures. Being a culturally responsive researcher involves the following: (a) explicit recognition, valuing, and discussion of cultural differences, (b) validation of the participants' world-view, (c) explicit discussion of power differentials, and (d) acknowledgment that non-traditional research methods may work better with participants of differing cultural values.

Relational ethics: This values dignity, mutual respect and connectedness between the researcher and researched, and between researchers and the communities they live and work in. Relational researchers balance their research with their obligations toward, care for, and connection with those who participate in their research.

Reflexive ethics: Researchers need to (a) be sensitive to the interactions of self, others and situations, (b) notice the reactions to a research situation and adapt in a responsive, ethical, moral way, where the participant's safety, privacy, dignity and autonomy are respected, (c) pay special attention to the possible power imbalances between the researcher and the participants, (d) use their writing and other forms of representation as a tool to be transparent so that that their work can be understood not only in terms of what was discovered, but how it was discovered.

As described above, a range of ethical positions are available to qualitative researchers. The alternative positions outlined make it clear that ethical issues are not over and done with, once ethical approval has been granted by the REC or an IRB. Institutional ethical approval is just the first step, the basic entry point, into a long and complex process. One reason for this is that doing research in the field can throw up an array of unexpected, subtle and nuanced ethical dilemmas that RECs and IRBs cannot control or predict. It is to the complexities of ethics as a *process* in the field, where researchers necessarily have to engage in an *ethics of practice*, or *situational ethics*, that we now turn our attention.

ethical issues in qualitative research

ETHICAL DILEMMAS IN THE FIELD

Informed consent

As outlined in Chapter 3, informed consent is based on the notion that people should be allowed to agree or refuse to participate in a study based on them having comprehensive information concerning the nature and purpose of the study. In a study by West, Bill and Martin (2010), which explored and compared research ethics processes and decisions within sport and exercise science departments and institutions, they found that 'informed consent was ranked as the most important ethical issue' (p. 150). Likewise, in health-related research, Franklin *et al.* (2012) argue that informed consent is at the heart of ethics because a researcher becomes 'informed about context-specific ethics through the questions and possible concerns that gatekeepers and the participants raise in the initial stages of a project' (p. 1731). They acknowledge, however, that seeking and gaining informed consent, particularly in organisational settings or where a number of stakeholders are involved, is no easy task. In some cases it is simply not possible, desirable, or safe to seek informed consent. Olive and Thorpe (2011) found this to be so when making observations from the chairlift of unidentifiable snowboarders and skiers interacting in the terrain park below them and when they attended a snowboarding event with thousands of young, intoxicated spectators.

Conducting covert research as described in Chapter 3 also means that informed consent is not sought from the participants involved in the study. Given the covert nature of the research role adopted, it is not possible to achieve informed consent without moving to an overt role which in many cases would undermine the purposes of the study. Consequently, as Lugosi (2006) notes, the covert researcher is sometimes accused of being deceitful, engaging in subterfuge, misleading people with whom they might interact, and thus doing 'unethical' research. For him, however, failing to gain informed consent when doing covert research does not mean researchers should necessarily stop conducting this form of inquiry. This is because there are many occasions when concealment is necessary, and often unavoidable.

An example of covert research that was deemed to be justifiable and in which informed consent was not sought can be found in the work of Pearson (2009). He undertook covert research with English football fans in order to study police responses to hooliganism. Pearson argued that overt research would not be an effective approach because, in interviews, while some fans exaggerated their involvement in illegal behaviours to present themselves as more exciting, those actually involved tended to downplay their involvement for fear of exposure. Furthermore, he wanted to witness police behaviour that he knew from experience could sometimes be abusive towards fans, but would be restrained if they knew they were being watched by an academic researcher from a university. In view of this, Pearson did not seek informed consent from either the football fans or the police. This was justified as the research was to be used by him to inform police practices in relation to the control of football crowds and, therefore, required that any feedback be based on spontaneous and un-staged events in the field.

Even when the researcher is overt and 'open' about the purposes of the study the process of gaining informed consent is not easy. Researchers most often seek informed consent from participants at the start of a study *before* the data collection has taken place and then at no point after. In this one-shot pre-study informed consent procedure, conversations about consent rarely extend beyond what occurs at the outset of a study. This assumes, as suggested in some traditional positions on ethics, that both the researcher and participant can predict how the research will unfold and what will happen in the weeks, months, and possibly years to come. This is simply not possible and raises questions about just how 'fully informed' participants can be at the start of a qualitative study given the emerging nature of this form of inquiry. For example, by its very nature conducting an ethnographic study is an emergent process of discovery that cannot be predicted in advance. As a consequence, any information provided to participants at the start of a study will be necessarily vague and contingent on what happens in the field as the study progresses.

Given such dilemmas, informed consent in qualitative research should not be seen as a singular event accomplished at the start of a study but rather as an ongoing process of construction and negotiation throughout the period of field work and beyond. Informed consent needs to be negotiated and re-established on a regular basis throughout a study with those involved. This *process consent* is consistent with the various aspirational ethical positions outlined earlier in this chapter.

An example of this approach in SEH is available in the life history work of Phoenix (2010a) with mature natural bodybuilders. Whilst Phoenix obtained written informed consent before the research started, she also

214

provided updates to the participants on how the project was unfolding throughout the study and she checked with them at various stages that they were still happy to be involved. Importantly, with those mature bodybuilders who agreed to take part in an auto-photography task as part of the study, Phoenix regularly checked with them that she could use the visual images they produced in publications, exhibitions and at conferences. In addition, Phoenix shared her written and visual analyses with her participants and discussed with them how they were 'interpreted' and represented. This 'member checking' was not done to validate interpretations or representations. Rather, it was done for reasons of engaging in process consent, which included entering into a dialogue with participants about ethical dilemmas that had arisen in the study and that might possibly emerge in the future.

Anonymity and confidentiality

In seeking to convince people to participate in their studies, qualitative researchers often offer the promise of anonymity. According to Walford (2005) anonymity simply means that 'we do not name the person or research site involved but, in research, it is usually extended to mean that we do not include information about any individual or research site that will enable the individual or research site to be identified by others' (p. 85). A number of research codes state that anonymity is a desirable standard in qualitative research, primarily as a means to ensure confidentiality and to minimise the risk of harm to participants (for example, British Sociological Association, 2002). For Kaiser (2009), the dominant approach to protecting participant confidentiality centres on making them unidentifiable in the belief that if participants remain anonymous it is less likely that harm will come their way.

Tilley and Woodthorpe (2011) acknowledge that, as a guiding principle of qualitative research, anonymity is a key ethical concept. They also acknowledge that it is a contested concept and has been the source of much academic discussion. For example, Wolcott (2002) argues that whilst we should not be opposed to keeping confidences and respecting the rights and privacy of those involved in our studies, it is important for qualitative researchers to recognise that they cannot 'think that such declarations can be made in absolute terms' (p. 147). Morse (2007) also advises against promising absolute confidentiality in the process of gaining consent as this can be very difficult to achieve in certain forms of qualitative inquiry. As

Tilley and Woodthorpe stress, however, there will always be qualitative research studies in which the anonymisation of participants is appropriate, for example, some research with children and vulnerable groups, research investigating highly sensitive topics, or research with participants for whom achieving informed consent may be a complex undertaking. They also note that anonymisation may be necessary when participants are in a complicated relationship with the researcher, for example, in the case of students that the researcher also teaches.

Against this, Tilley and Woodthorpe (2011) ask the following questions: Where does this leave the researcher who wants to identify their sites and/or participants? Of the participants who want to be identified? What of those researchers who feel they *have* to identify their research sites and/or participants? They also point out that there may be times when the principle of anonymity conflicts with the aims of the research, the dissemination activity, and with the researcher's obligations to be accountable to funders and engage in knowledge transfer.

Often RECs and IRBs formalise anonymity as a methodological given in their written guidelines. This is particularly problematic for those conducting ethnographies, or undertaking life history, narrative work or case study research and for those committed to openly ideological forms of inquiry that are participatory or emancipatory in nature.

> On the one hand, to reveal identifying features challenges the normal expectation of the benefit of protection that anonymity brings; on the other, upholding the principle of autonomy could actually serve to undermine the research and/or participants' autonomy. In particular, where participants are active agents in the research – as they can be with participatory or emancipatory approaches – there is a strong case to be made for offering individuals and organizations the choice as to whether or not their identities are disclosed, even if this may create conflict between participants' and researchers' autonomy.
>
> (Tilley & Woodthorpe, 2011: 200)

Kaiser (2009) points out that many participants in qualitative studies can feel a sense of 'losing ownership' of the data when it becomes anonymised in the dissemination process. This issue of data ownership becomes extremely important in those forms of research where the central purpose of the study is to 'give voice' to previously silenced or marginalised individuals and groups. In view of all this, Tilley and Wood-thorpe (2011) believe the expectation that anonymity should be maintained throughout the research process and at the point of dissemination, 'can serve to create further ethical challenges when research sites and their participants are "dislodged from their histories and geographies"' (p. 200).

It is also important to recognise the gulf between the 'promise' of anonymity and the 'reality' of practice. This is particularly so given the need for 'good' qualitative studies to provide rich description and contextual data of events, individuals, and the practices of groups so that the reader can engage with the world through the senses of the participants and, for example, make naturalistic generalisations to others situations (see Chapter 6). In so doing, the participants necessarily become recognisable to themselves and to others. To emphasise the dilemma, consider what qualitative research would look like if this was not the case. Imagine an ethnographic study of a sports club in transition, or a life history study of injured athletes, in which the participants *do not* recognise themselves, key events, and social practices in the final report. Such an outcome would raise serious questions about the quality of the qualitative study.

Even if pseudonyms are used and place names changed and so on, the 'better' a qualitative study is the 'worse' it is at maintaining the anonymity of the participant and the setting. This is particularly so when the study focuses on one individual, one club, or one particular setting. It is even more so if any of these are members of an elite that is already known to the public. As Mellick and Fleming (2010) comment, 'The very public (and publicized) nature of elite level sport can, however, create tensions for narrative accounts when other actors *are* central. In particular, the researcher's attempts to observe recognized good practice in research ethics can be troublesome' (p. 300). In their own case study of referee communication in rugby football union that focused on one referee's encounters with three key 'actors' (his mentor, a club coach, and a player – with a rich and detailed biography), Mellick and Fleming faced extreme difficulties in providing a rich narrative account whilst attempting to protect anonymity. For example, disclosed identity was almost inevitable with the rugby player involved because he was the former national team captain who retired from the Australian squad which probably makes him a 'unique case study'.

The dilemma for Mellick and Flemming (2010) was that the biography of the player was crucial to the narrative they wanted to craft. Also the fact that the player had captained Australia and had a reputation among referees that preceded him was central to the expectancy theory that shaped the conceptual underpinning of a later study that Mellick was to conduct. As such, to 'remove that aspect of the narrative would render it impotent' (p. 307). Similarly, in their narrative study of an elite athlete's experience of cancer, Sparkes, Pérez-Samaniego *et al.* (2012) and the participant recognised from the start that even if they used a pseudonym and changed place names, given his public profile as an athlete who had won major competitions and been diagnosed with cancer which was reported in newspapers, that it would be impossible to achieve 'total' anonymity and it would be easy for interested parties to identify him.

The same could be said with regard to issues of *confidentiality* that goes hand-in-hand with the notion of anonymity and which is also a promise often made by qualitative researchers. In this regard, Kaiser (2009) speaks of *deductive disclosure*, also known as *internal confidentiality*. This occurs when the traits of individuals or groups make them identifiable in research reports. For him, given that qualitative studies often contain rich descriptions of study participants, 'confidentiality breaches via deductive disclosure are a particular concern for qualitative researchers. As such, qualitative researchers face a conflict between conveying detailed, accurate accounts of the social world and protecting the identities of the individuals who participated in their research' (p. 1632).

Others have also noted the dilemmas of conducting rigorous qualitative research and protecting confidentiality. This is particularly so with regard to what Damianakis and Woodford (2012) call *small connected communities* that are geographically bound and tightly knit (for example, a sports club, team, or organisation). In studies of these communities, the possibility for unintentional identity disclosure is magnified; 'such identification is also possible when participants know each other through connections that transcend shared geography, such as, professional or personal networks (for example, professional associations or online health support groups' (p. 709). As with attempts to maintain anonymity, attempts to maintain confidentiality often involve the use of pseudonyms instead of real names, and changing place names and location is necessarily limited in its ability to succeed. As Kaiser (2009) notes regarding this process of *data cleaning*, although researchers can be meticulous in this task 'the contextual identifiers in individuals' life stories will remain. This is particularly true for respondents who have faced unusual life events or who are unique in some way' (p. 1635).

Kaiser (2009) suggests that in presenting the life story of participants that researchers need to consider whether the specific quotations and examples they include when disseminating their findings could lead to their participants being identified via deductive disclosure, and also whether it might lead to those associated with the participants being identified (for example, teammates, coaches and family members). For her, this might mean that the data will need to be modified in some way. Of course, it is the researcher who takes responsibility for deciding what aspects of a person's stories or life circumstances need to be changed to maintain confidentiality. This will vary from researcher to researcher depending on the case in question. Modifying empirical data in qualitative research, however, raises another issue for Kaiser in that, unlike changing a specific name, 'changing additional details to render data unidentifiable can alter or destroy the original meaning of the data' (p. 1635).

Within sport studies, similar points are made by Mellick and Fleming (2010) who observed that when rich descriptions are 'toned down' to protect anonymity and confidentiality in qualitative research this strategy can render the written report 'less authentic and the analysis less persuasive' (p. 301). Reflecting on a study that focused on a rugby union football referee's encounter with three key 'actors' they highlighted another dilemma that cleaning the data can lead to which involves the case of *mistaken identity*. This is more likely to occur when the case study is not unique but relatively unusual and when additional disguise is also added. As Mellick and Fleming note, 'when some details are omitted and/or when spurious detail is included to conceal the identity, it is possible to implicate another person altogether' (p. 308). In their study, they suggest that one of their key actors, the mentor, may have been such an example. That is, the description provided of him is such that readers may infer incorrectly that it is someone else entirely.

In addition, Kaiser (2009) notes that readers are typically unaware of how data has been altered and are, therefore, 'unable to consider the significance of changes for their interpretations of the data or for the validity of the data' (p. 1635). Little is known about how participants in studies might feel and respond to having their data altered and the meanings of what they said and did compromised. Corden and Sainsbury (2006), however, report that participants often have strong feelings about how their words or their personal characteristics are altered in research reports. This links to the point made by Kaiser that not only might a participant object to such data cleaning, they might also object to *not* being named in the final reports. It should not, therefore, be assumed that everyone in the study wants complete confidentiality. Of course, honouring the desire to be named by one participant raises other ethical issues about disclosing the identity of those closely associated with them, such as, family members, team mates or coaches.

Issues of anonymity and confidentiality are crystallised in qualitative research that utilises visual methods. Here, Phoenix (2010a) talks of a moral maze and notes there is limited agreement amongst ethics committees and visual researchers on ethical guidelines and resultant practices. Likewise, with regard to *sociological photographers*, Harper (2005) highlights the ethical dilemmas associated with informed consent, subject anonymity and confidentiality when the photographing of public life is central to the research process and where, often, 'the identifiability of subjects is critical to the sociological usefulness of the images; these include elements such as subjects' expressions, gestures, hairstyles, clothing, and other personal attributes' (p. 760).

In accordance with process ethics such issues need to be made clear at the start of the study and then discussed throughout. Participants should be fully involved in any decision to use visual data in the dissemination process. In this regard, the British Sociological Association Visual Sociology Study Group statement on ethics is a useful starting point for dealing with such issues. The following are some of the points they raise regarding of the use of photography in research studies:

- When using participants' own photographs, the researcher(s) should make the participant aware that, as creators of images, they (the image-makers(s)) are legally the owners. Thus the researcher(s) must have the participants' permission to use the photographs in publication (including publications on websites).
- Researchers may want to discuss the status of the images with participants in order to clearly explain the dissemination strategy of the research project. In certain circumstances, the researcher(s) may want to create a written or verbal contract guaranteeing the participants ownership of the images produced. Under UK law copyright can be waived by participants and given to the researcher(s); however it is recommended that researchers read the current legislation or seek legal advice if taking this option (please note that the date of the creation of the image affects the legal status).

220

- In the use of archives or participants' own photo albums it is important to make clear your intended use of the document and obtain the relevant permissions to use the image.
- Images depicting illegal activities, including criminal damage, sexual violence and hate crime do not have the privilege of confidentiality.
- Visual data which at one point may have been everyday can become extremely sensitive; in such instances members should not put the publication of the research before the physical, social and psychological well-being of participants.
- Members should note that in various cultures, certain visual research methods may offend the research setting and participants. For instance; the use of photo-documentary in aboriginal communities, or the use of write-and-draw techniques to explore notions of deity in Islamic communities. In these cases the researcher(s) should subject the research strategy to a high level of critical scrutiny and seek advice or comment from a professionally recognised ethics board. Issues that may arise include risks of censorship, threats to freedom of academic speech and offending a community.
- Sociologists should be careful, on the one hand, not to give unrealistic guarantees of confidentiality and, on the other, not to permit communication of research films or records to audiences other than those to which the research participants have agreed.

(Source: www.visualsociology.org.uk/about/
ethical_statement.php)

Beyond visual sociology, others have also suggested strategies for qualitative researchers to deal with issue of anonymity and confidentiality. Kaiser (2009) offers a number of recommendations that revolve around making the participants better informed of the use of the data (that is, who the audience is for the study results and how the study results will be disseminated), and facilitating dialogue with participants about how their data can be used (that is, revising the informed consent process). With regard to determining audience and dissemination plans, Kaiser notes that every project has a number of potential audiences, and that results can be shared via different kinds of presentation. These need to be discussed with participants throughout the study so that the implications for whether or not confidentiality and anonymity is possible or, indeed, desirable can be negotiated. Of course, while it is not feasible to predict every potential audience due to the emergent nature of qualitative inquiry, the responsibility lies with the researcher to carefully consider future data use. If the data leads, however, to different forms of dissemination that were not anticipated during the study then, as Kaiser argues, the participants should be re-contacted to gain their permission to use their data in these unanticipated ways.

Kaiser (2009) also suggests that researchers need to acknowledge that the participants themselves are an audience for the findings. Accordingly, the findings and interpretations of the researcher should be made available to the participants at various stages of the study in order to solicit feedback from them. This precludes any assumption that all the participants want confidentiality and to remain anonymous. Further, it does not assume that the participants will allow the researcher to take sole responsibility for editing and cleaning data to ensure these outcomes are achieved. Rather, issues of confidentiality and anonymity become part of an ongoing dialogue between researchers and participants to determine if they wish to remain anonymous or if they wish to be identified in the research. Such an approach, Kaiser notes, is reflected in the ethical guidelines of the American Anthropological Association that expect anthropological researchers to determine in advance whether their host or providers of information wish to remain anonymous or receive recognition, and then make every effort to comply with these wishes. These guidelines also make it clear that researchers must present to their research participants the possible impact of the choices, and make clear that despite their best efforts, anonymity may be compromised or recognition fail to materialise. Hewitt (2007) agrees and makes the case that when interviewing, ground rules about confidentiality should be established with participants. This being particularly so when there is risk that participants' disclosures may reveal potentially 'significant harm to self or others, which would require that confidentiality be overridden, or when political control over the dissemination of findings might not be within the researcher's control' (p. 1155).

The ongoing dialogue about confidentiality and anonymity proposed by Kaiser (2009) has implications for the informed consent process which might need to be modified according to the outcomes of the dialogue between participants and researcher. For her, a re-envisioned informed consent process should include greater detail about the audience for one's research, be ongoing, and present participants with a wider range of confidentiality options. To provide this wider range of options, Kaiser argues that a more nuanced view of consent is required, moving away from the assumption that every participant desires complete confidentiality, and moving towards understanding that a research participant might want to receive some recognition for some or all of what he or she contributes. She warns that if it is assumed that all study participants want complete confidentiality the 'researchers risk becoming paternalistic and denying participants their voice and the freedom to choose how their data is handled' (p. 1638).

Another strategy that can be discussed with participants is the form of representation used to describe them and others involved in the study (see Chapter 6). For example, the use of vignettes to present research or the use of composite characters is a possibility, as well as the use of creative nonfiction stories as these use 'real' data in ways that can maintain the anonymity and confidentiality of the participants whilst still providing rich description of people, events and processes. Alternatively, interview data might be transformed into a poetic representation for ethical purposes. Such an example is provided by Sparkes and Douglas (2007) who decided to portray the experiences of one elite female golf professional in their study in poetic form as opposed to the more traditional realist tale they told about the other six elite golfers that were interviewed. They chose this strategy because this golfer shared 'secret knowledge' with them about 'throwing' major games in professional tournaments. For Sparkes and Douglas, this secret knowledge raised ethical dilemmas about how best to represent her experiences and how to maintain the participant's anonymity when the stakes for her were high if anyone could identify her in the research. This strategy was discussed with the participant during the study who agreed this was the best option in her case. She also read the poetic representations that were produced based on her own words and acknowledged that whilst they captured the essence of her experiences they also maintained her anonymity.

A number of strategies are available for qualitative researchers in SEH to deal with issues of informed consent, anonymity and confidentiality. As indicated above, whilst addressing these issues is a necessary first step in gaining ethical clearance for RECs and IRBs, there are many steps beyond this moment. In keeping with the notion of aspirational ethics as an ongoing process of construction and negotiation, a dialogue about informed consent, anonymity and confidentiality needs to be maintained throughout the study and beyond for all those involved.

RESEARCH AS THERAPY

Various forms of qualitative research, such as life history and narrative studies, involve extended periods of one-to-one interaction between the researcher and the participant where the latter tells their story in their own words and at their own pace. As indicated in Chapter 4, the researcher is an active and attentive but non-judgmental listener in this interviewing process. Here, the personal, constitutive and reflective nature of sharing stories, the cathartic power of talking about experiences, and the fact that another person (that is the researcher) is empathetically listening and attending to (often) previously unspoken tales can have a powerful impact on the interviewee as storyteller (Hart & Crawford-Wright, 1999; Morse, 2007). This is particularly so when, over time, rapport and trust are built up between the researcher and the participant who may venture to explore deeply personal and emotional issues during the interview that can lead to a range of outcomes for the interviewee that can include greater self-understanding and opportunities for personal growth.

As Bondi (2013) points out, a number of qualitative researchers have observed that research activities such as participating in research interviews is 'sometimes beneficial for participants in ways that might reasonably be described as therapeutic' (p. 10). She continues as follows:

> The invitation to talk in this way in the presence of an interested and attentive listener may be very welcome to research participants; indeed, it may be the motivating factor for their participation. Because talking openly and telling one's stories is also associated with what clients do in psychotherapeutic settings, however, it is not surprising that researchers and participants sometimes feel confused and uncertain about what is happening and what is appropriate within research interviews. This has generated concern about the ethical responsibilities of researchers to participants who might find themselves unwittingly drawn into something far more like psychotherapy than they had anticipated ... That research interviews might be welcomed by participants as therapeutic opportunities is certainly no surprise.
>
> (Bondi, 2013: 10)

Set against this, participants may find themselves confronting difficult personal and psychological issues in such interviews. Sharing their stories could result in feelings of anxiety, distress, or guilt that can impact negatively on their well-being. With empathy, trust and rapport, he or she can also become emotionally reliant on the researcher. This poses the additional dilemma of how the researcher might leave the field in an ethically informed and caring manner. Providing the opportunity for another to tell a story about significant events in qualitative research can, therefore, have both positive and negative consequences.

Given these conditions, RECs and IRBs are often rightly concerned that some kind of therapy might be taking place and that the researcher might be adopting a therapeutic role during the interaction. There are, indeed, similarities between talk-based qualitative forms of inquiry and therapy. Equally, there are important differences that need to be acknowledged.

In terms of similarities, Bondi (2013) notes that qualitative research and psychotherapy are both projects of *making meaning*. For her, those participating in psychotherapy engage in processes of meaning-making within a psychiatric frame while those participating in research are invited to tell and perhaps explore their stories in a research frame. The attentive and active listening provided by the researcher is also similar to that of the psychotherapist. Likewise, when researchers meet with participants recurrently, relationships develop further, which can make it similar to psychotherapy or perhaps more akin to becoming friends. As Bondi points out, in all these cases, in various ways, when research participants tell their stories to attentive listeners, 'the act of narration in the presence of sympathetic witnesses is likely to enable participants to hear themselves anew in ways that make their stories freshly meaningful to themselves as well as for the researchers listening to them' (p. 11).

While qualitative researchers and psychotherapy may share a commitment to making meaning, Bondi (2013) is quick to point out that the meanings they make take different forms and circulate in different ways.

> For researchers the new personal meanings arising for research participants are not their sole purpose and not usually even their core purpose. Furthermore, new personal meanings in and of themselves do not generally constitute the research. Instead, however important these meanings might be, they also need to be put into wider circulation.
>
> (Bondi, 2013: 11)

For Bondi, in qualitative inquiry, researchers work, often in collaboration with their participants, with the materials they and their participants generate *beyond* their initial encounters to develop explicitly articulated, convincing and persuasive arguments or stories. She notes that these arguments or stories, which typically anonymise research participants, are made widely available through conferences, seminars and publications. Indeed, Bondi agues, 'it is only when ideas and arguments are communicated and disseminated that they become the stuff of research and scholarship' (p. 11).

In contrast, Bondi (2013) emphasises that in psychotherapy 'what matters is that the client or patient senses, feels or embodies something meaningful and generative. This 'something' is elusive and often implicit' (p. 11). Furthermore, given the nature of the engagement, one of the challenges that therapists face in communicating about their work outside tightly drawn professional boundaries is that the meanings generated 'are not ordinarily available for us to use *for any purpose beyond the therapeutic relationship*' (p. 11, emphasis added).

> Qualitative research seeks to make new meanings for particular forms of public circulation but often also enables more personal meaning making for those involved as participants and researchers. In psychotherapy, meaning making operates via the personal level and circulates primarily through how lives are lived . . . I would argue that confidentiality is a prerequisite for psychotherapy while publication of some kind is a requirement for research. Consequently, routes into publicly circulating discourses take different forms.
>
> (Bondi, 2013: 12)

Despite these differences in purpose, intent, forms and modes of circulation between researchers and research interviews and psychotherapists and the therapeutic encounter, it remains that any social situation involving prolonged interaction in a supportive environment can be defined as an *occasion for therapy* by one or more of the parties involved. Therefore, *unintentional* 'therapy' may occur in many sets of circumstances. As Hart and Crawford-Wright (2007) emphasise, however, there is a difference between a research interview and a therapy session in that 'in the former the participant is helping the researcher, whereas in the latter the therapist is helping the client. Therefore, it is not possible for one to become the other without the motivations of the players changing dramatically' (p. 206). Similarly, Morse (2007) argues that researchers need to be reflexive of the dangers of confusing research with therapy. For her,

226

the purposes behind these and the goals between the two are very different, and these differences need to be respected.

Acknowledging that most researchers are not professionally qualified therapists but recognising the dangers that they might be perceived as such by participants, Hewitt (2007) recommends that researchers carefully clarify their purposes and role compared to therapists and continue this process of clarification throughout the study. This might begin with the simple statement, 'Please note, I am a researcher interested in your life story and experiences but I am not a qualified therapist. Before we start, I would like to make the differences between the two clear so that you are better able to understand the purpose of my study and our roles during the interviews we will have together'. Equally, when sometimes participants joke that they are enjoying the 'therapy' sessions (that is, the interviews), the researcher can use this as a light-hearted occasion to remind them that they are not therapists and to once again clarify their roles.

Besides this ongoing process of clarification, researchers can also ensure they have contact details to facilitate the onward referral of research participants to professional sources of support should issues and reactions arise during the interviews that are beyond the remit and capabilities of the researcher. Likewise, these professional sources could be used to debrief participants at the end of the study. To this end, Bondi (2013) suggests that researchers need to have adequate training and support which may include the use of group psychotherapy or research-focused therapeutic supervisions as part of a self-care strategy for the researcher. This is an important point as the impact of the interview process on the researcher, especially when they are dealing with traumatic issues such as career-ending injury or sexual abuse in sport can be upsetting and disturbing. In short, researchers are vulnerable subjects too and like the participants in their study need to be treated with an ethic of care by themselves and others.

This is not to say that when the researcher is a professionally qualified therapist that tensions and ethical dilemmas are resolved. Herzog and Hays (2012) who are both licensed health practitioners, address the challenging conundrum of when to offer psychotherapy versus mental skills training by describing four actual cases that illustrate the different ways in which clients present and practitioners respond. They begin by articulating a practice continuum that ranges from psychotherapy to mental skills training in which counselling occupies the middle ground.

Broadly speaking, Herzog and Hays consider 'psychotherapy' to involve the 'psychological treatment of (diagnosed or diagnosable) mental or emotional disorders, to assist in relief from symptoms, return to previous functioning, or improve daily functioning' (p. 487). In contrast, mental skills training or coaching, rests on the assumption that the client has 'sufficient mental strength to be able to profit from an educational focus on particular skills that will enhance performance' (p. 488). In between these, is counselling that involves the work of helping people to cope with everyday problems and opportunities. This encompasses more aspects of therapy than mental skills training.

For Herzog and Hays (2012), even though the distinctions between psychotherapy and counselling are valid at a *theoretical* level, they stress that in *actuality*, the distinction may be imperceptible, 'a function of the practitioner's training, designation, and practice orientation; the practice setting; and the client's interests, preferences, and goals' (p. 488). The ways that boundaries can blur between psychotherapy, counselling and mental skills training are illustrated by the four case studies that Herzog and Hays present that involve (1) mental skills training shifting to therapy; (2) therapeutic work shifting to mental skills training; (3) simultaneous work between two practitioners, and (4) alternating services from the same practitioner. In reflecting on these cases they note that the 'balance and shift between psychotherapy and mental skills training is often complex; practitioners need to be knowledgeable and versatile; often, there is no one right solution but rather, many potential paths' (p. 495). For them, as practitioners with proper licensure navigate along the psychotherapy–mental skills training continuum and engage with the four basic configurations as described, they are 'well-advised to do so with thoughtfulness and care throughout the process' (p. 498).

THE INTERNET

The increasing and widespread use of the internet provides new vantage points from which to observe conventional behaviour and view new kinds of behaviour, as well as provide new tools with which to gain access to a diverse range of data. Not surprisingly, the internet is increasingly becoming a rich data source for qualitative researchers. At one level, reaping the wealth of data 'out there' on the internet would appear to be non-problematic. Using the internet as a researcher brings with it a number of ethical dilemmas, however. These can be particularly difficult to navigate due to the rapid changes in internet technology and the ways in which this is accessed and manipulated by various user groups. As a consequence, what might not be a problem today could be tomorrow. The situation is well described in the 'Description and Scope' statement of the *International Journal of Internet Research Ethics* that was launched in 2008. This statement raises questions about what happens when 'populations', locales and spaces that previously had no corresponding physical environment become a focal point, or site of research activity:

> Human subjects' protections questions then began to arise, across disciplines and over time: What about privacy? How is informed consent obtained? What about research on minors? What are 'harms' in an online environment? Is this really human subject's work? More broadly, are the ethical obligations of researchers conducting research online somehow different from other forms of research ethics practices? . . . How do diverse *methodological* approaches result in distinctive ethical conflicts – and, possibly, distinctive ethical resolutions? How do diverse *cultural* and *legal* traditions shape what are perceived as ethical conflicts and permissible resolutions? How do researchers collaborating across diverse ethical and legal domains recognize and resolve ethical issues in ways that recognize and incorporate often markedly different ethical understandings? . . . Such questions are at the heart of IRE scholarship, and such general areas as anonymity, privacy, ownership, authorial ethics, legal issues, research ethics principles (justice, beneficence, respect for persons), and consent are appropriate areas for consideration.

Regarding internet research ethics, Buchanan and Zimmer (2012) note that there is little research that is not impacted in some way on or through the internet. As such, the internet, as a field, a tool and a venue, brings up specific and far-reaching ethical issues. They point out that as the internet has evolved into a more social and communicative tool and venue, the ethical issues have shifted from purely data-driven to more human-centred concerns. 'On-ground' or face-to-face analogies, therefore, may not be applicable to online research. For example, the concept of the public park has been used as a site where researchers can observe others, but online, the concepts of public and private are much more complex. As a result of all of this, Buchanan and Zimmer state that RECs and IRBs have been confronted with a series of new ethical issues that include the following questions:

- What ethical obligations do researchers have to protect the privacy of subjects engaging in activities in 'public' internet spaces?
- How is confidentiality or anonymity assured online?
- How is and should informed consent be obtained online?
- How should research on minors be conducted, and how do you prove a subject is not a minor?
- Is deception (pretending to be someone you are not, withholding identifiable information, and so on) online a norm or a harm?
- How is 'harm' possible to someone existing in an online space?

Given that the ethics of internet research is an emerging field, readers are directed to specialist journals on this topic, such as, the *International Journal of Internet Research Ethics,* and specialist books, such as, *The Ethics of Internet Research: A Rhetorical, Case-Based Process* by McKee and Porter (2009). This book provides a comprehensive overview of regulatory frameworks and national and international law relevant to internet research. It also presents a range of case studies that document the variety of ethical challenges facing internet researchers in diverse contexts and settings along with the multiple strategies and practices they have brought into play in efforts to resolve these challenges.

To give a flavour of what is involved in internet ethics, we now focus on but one of these that revolves around what constitutes 'private' and 'public' data in this domain. Do researchers examining blogs need to gain authorial permission from bloggers when recording their posts? Is blog material academic 'fair game' or is informed consent needed? If so, is it possible to obtain consent? Is an invasion of privacy possible concerning items in the public domain?

There are no straightforward answers to such questions. This is because no consensus exists among researchers concerning how to deal with the ethics associated with what is public or private. Despite considerable variation, Hookway (2008) notes that responses to the broader question of what is private and what is public online tend to fall into one of three positions. Position One proposes that archived material on the internet is publicly available, academic 'fair-game', and 'therefore participant consent is not necessary' (p. 105). Advocates of this position tend to make the following case:

Blogs are firmly located in the public domain and for this reason it can be argued that the necessity of consent should be waived. Further, blogs are public not only in the sense of being publicly accessible . . . but also in how they are defined by users. Blogging is a public act of writing for an implicit audience. The exception proves the rule: blogs that are interpreted by bloggers as 'private' are made 'friends only'. Thus, accessible blogs may be personal but they are not private.

(Hookway, 2008: 105)

In contrast, as Hookway (2008) notes, Position Two claims 'that online postings, though publicly accessible, are written with an expectation of privacy and should be treated as such' (p. 105). Against this, Position Three holds the view that online interaction 'defies clear-cut prescription as either public or private' (p. 105). The boundaries between public and private are blurred. The internet can be seen as a place where what people do is simultaneously publicly private and privately public. As such, how actors themselves define their participation in online environments might be the most important issue that researchers need to address.

With regard to making an ethical application to a REC or an IRB, researchers need to adopt a position regarding their use of the internet even though this position might change over time. The position initially adopted will shape what data is collected (if any) and how it is collected. To help with this, and ethics in general on the internet, a very useful resource is *The Association of Internet Researchers*, who published their own set of ethical guidelines, authored by Markham and Buchanan (2012). These guidelines offer a set of questions to prompt reflection about ethical decision-making within the specific confines of one's study.

A number of the issues mentioned above have been touched upon by researchers within SEH who have used the internet as a resource for gathering data. Griggs (2011) discussed the ethics of consent, deception, privacy and confidentiality in relation to the use of the internet as a method of data collection within the alternative sporting subculture of Ultimate Frisbee. Another example can be found in Smith and Stewart's (2012) study of the social constructions, body perceptions and health experiences of a serious recreational competitive bodybuilder and powerlifter community. Data were obtained over a period of thirty-six months from a discussion forum appearing within an online community dedicated to muscular development.

Although participants in their study employed 'avatar' names as pseudonyms, Smith and Stewart decided for ethical reasons to change participant identities in the written results of the research. The stanzas or lines of coded posts they collected, however, were reproduced exactly without corrections, editing, or censorship. Further, consistent with university protocols they 'did not make personal contact with participants, as the research could be undertaken without risk or harm on a nonvulnerable community, where a posted site policy notified users of its public access . . . We therefore maintained a purely observational status wherein we played the roles of specialised "lurkers"' (p. 974).

In addition to the ethical dilemmas signalled above, qualitative researchers who are considering doing internet research also need to be aware of the copyright laws pertaining to their countries. As Hookway (2008) notes, in Australia, the UK and the USA, internet content is automatically copyrighted. This means that the moment certain entries, like a blog entry, are uploaded onto a content management system they are protected by copyright. Bloggers, therefore, like many other internet users, have exclusive rights over the reproduction of their work. It is always conceivable, then, that a user might not grant a researcher the rights to reproduce their work in a thesis, journal article, or book. Given this, any researcher using internet data must carefully consider before, during, and after conducting the study if what is put on the internet can be reproduced in the research they will write up. Failure to gain permission from the blogger or someone else could mean their work cannot be published.

Clearly, for qualitative researchers the internet raises many ethical dilemmas and challenges. These revolve around how to balance collecting, analysing and representing internet data with disciplinary, institutional, legal and cultural ethical obligations and aspirations. Before doing internet research it is therefore important for the qualitative researcher to engage with the ethical dilemmas and challenges that accompany it. This is especially so as the technologies themselves change rapidly. As always, then, the decision-making process to do internet research needs to be informed and, as part of this, include a concern with the process of ethics.

232

PROTECTING THE RESEARCHER

Just as participants need protecting, so do researchers. This point is too often overlooked. As Morse (2007) states, 'Safety of the researcher is one of the least addressed yet most important considerations in qualitative inquiry' (p. 1005). For her, this is not just about physical safety of researchers, but also about the care of the emotional self.

> Therefore, we must recognize the influence of the research topic on one's self and one's emotional well-being, and provide support and debriefing for the entire research team. This is essential and needed both during data collection and when working with data, including writing up.
>
> (Morse, 2007: 1005)

Sugden (2012) suggests that ethnography is inherently perilous, and that the risks multiply when the (under) worlds you set out to access and share are at the margins of society and those that you research have something to hide. Reflecting on various projects he recalls being threatened with extreme violence as well as with legal action by sports organisations.

> However, the level of risk can be minimized. The most important thing is for the researcher to be acutely aware that once in the field he or she is always at risk. In order to maximize understanding, fieldworkers should be ever alert to what is going on around them. To achieve this, they need to develop highly tuned 'sociological antenna': using and extending our natural abilities to be acutely aware of what is going on at the centre, periphery and every corner of the social milieu that we find ourselves in. This is required for the generation of data, but it is also essential for self-preservation.
>
> (Sugden, 2012: 249)

For Sugden (2012) researchers need to make judgements in the field about when it is safe to stay and when it is the time to leave. An escape route is required. He does not favour fully covert research, as entering the field and posing as somebody else to all participants, including gatekeepers, offers no protection should the true identity of the researcher become known. In his various studies, if he had been fully covert, Sugden suggests, no one at all in the field would have known he was a researcher, and thus he would have been left at major risk. When somebody in the field (for example the gatekeeper) who could provide some protection knew he was a researcher, however, then Sugden was provided with a legitimate excuse for not doing certain things and had an escape route out of certain settings – a 'get out of jail free' card.

Less dramatic, but no less important, is the need for emotional as well as physical self-care in the field. Exploring the experiences of others can be emotionally draining and at times disturbing, especially when dealing with traumatic events. Here, a good example is provided in the work of Brewer and Sparkes (2011) in their ethnographic study of how young people experienced parental death and the role of physical activity in the process of coping with this event. As Jo Brewer herself had experienced parental bereavement at the age of fifteen, and been supported by the charity (The Rocky Centre) that was the site for the ethnography, the emotional dynamics of interviewing other parentally bereaved young people and being involved as a full participant in various activities with them, was an issue of self-care from the start.

Jo noted in her field diary that she often came away from interviews feeling inspired and euphoric. On other occasions she left interviews feeling anxious and disturbed. Sometimes the effect of the interview on her was delayed. For example, the day after conducting one interview that had a powerful impact on her, Jo recognised, as she reflected back on the interview while transcribing it, that she experienced three clear manifestations of embodied stress in the form of bad chest pains, a lingering headache, and then a nosebleed. In her field diary she notes that she felt really tired and ended up going to bed early: 'It was as if the process of transcribing the interview had physically and emotionally drained me'. Given the nature of this kind of work, the cumulative effects of continued emotional engagement and challenges in the field need to be considered and appropriate support provided as part of an ethic of care. Accordingly, beyond the regular meetings Jo had with her supervisor (Andrew Sparkes) that included both 'academic' and 'emotional' support, arrangements were made for Jo to meet on a regular basis with a qualified clinical psychologist who worked at the Rocky Centre and who had personally known her for ten years. These meetings provided Jo with the opportunity to discuss any feelings the research may have triggered in her and be provided with appropriate emotional support throughout the study.

Too often, self-care within qualitative projects is left to the researchers themselves. This is evident in the work of Sparkes and Smith (2012a) who, in making the case that narrative analysis involves an embodied engagement with the lives of others, explore some of the reactions they experienced in their life history study of amateur rugby players who suffered a spinal cord injury and became disabled through playing this sport. Extracts are provided from Brett's field diary about his reactions to an interview he conducted with a participant called Jamie who told a particularly harrowing, anxiety-provoking and chaotic story that disturbed Brett both within and beyond the interview setting (Smith & Sparkes, 2008). This is followed by Andrew's reactions to the visible impact the interview has on Brett and how he tried to assist him cope with the situation.

For the most part, as Dickson-Swift, James, Kippen and Liamputtong, (2007) note when considering the emotional work undertaken in sensitive qualitative research and the kinds of support made available to researchers, this tends to be accomplished on an informal basis. That is, researchers tend to use informal support networks of colleagues, trusted friends, and family members for support and debriefing throughout their research. Dickson-Swift and colleagues acknowledge a growing acceptance among qualitative researchers that they might need some therapeutic support to deal with issues that arise from their inquiries into sensitive topics. Just what kind of therapeutic support might be required and how it should be used is worthy of further discussion by the qualitative research community in SEH.

SUMMARY

In this chapter we have outlined a number of ethical positions that qualitative researchers in SEH might adopt. We have noted the differences between what might be described as procedural ethics and process ethics. For us, while issues relating to procedural ethics are foregrounded as a pre-study task framed by applications to RECs and IRBs, there is a rapid shift to process ethics on entry to the messy realities of the field. We illustrated this by considering the complexities of informed consent, anonymity and confidentiality in relation to qualitative research. Following this we focused on the tensions revolving around the issue of 'research as therapy'. Finally, we considered the ethical dilemmas of using the internet as a data resource and the protection of researchers.

At various points we have noted the problems that qualitative researchers can encounter in their dealings with IRBs and RECS, and have commented on their limitations to deal with the ethical dilemmas that might occur in the field. Like Tolich (2010) we recognise that the qualitative researcher is repeatedly subjected to 'unjust' scrutiny by IRBs and RECs and that this state of affairs often leads to qualitative researchers keeping 'their heads below the ethical parapet, reluctant to comment on their own practice for fear of giving IRBs more grist for the mill' (p. 1608). Despite this we are not advocating a rejection of minimalist codes of ethics or the abolition of RECs or IRBs. We would recommend these as resources to be used by qualitative researchers to reflect on specific ethical issues. Like Lahman *et al.* (2011), in light of the unpredictable nature of human research that does not allow researchers to anticipate all consequences, we do feel that 'additional considerations that cannot and should not be regulated are necessary for ethical research practice' (p. 1399).

Rather than qualitative researchers keeping their heads below the ethical parapet, we concur with Ellis (2007) who recommends that qualitative researchers need to better communicate their study design and research plans to IRBs and RECs. Research teams need to refine their skills to explain procedures relating to qualitative methods prior to data gathering. This communication should include a description of the uncertainties that are part of qualitative inquiry, and an explanation that unforeseeable situations are likely to arise in the field. In response, Ellis hopes that IRBs and RECs will begin to adopt an open, exploratory attitude towards inductive research proposals. Here, researchers would have the opportunity to argue their case and present it in a coherent form within the field of qualitative inquiry without having to employ quantitative research measures and templates.

In the case of successful communication between qualitative researchers and an IRB or REC, Franklin *et al.* (2012) suggest that 'the accumulation of examples and experiences, and establishment of common ground could lead to a situation in which the board can shift from being a disciplining institution to a stakeholder in the process' (p. 1730). They also support the view that qualitative researchers need to invest more time in 'educating' members of IRBs and RECs so that a common understanding is developed regarding what can be expected from a qualitative proposal. Franklin and her colleagues do not wish to disparage the expertise of such members. They do however emphasise that, well intentioned though RECs and IRBs are, their members are not necessarily the best people to decide on the risks and benefits of various forms of qualitative research.

236

Beyond all of this, Wolcott (2010) emphasises that ultimately, the responsibility for what we do, say, and reveal remains, as it must, only with ourselves. He concludes as follows:

> Anyone who has ever taught qualitative methods realizes that it would be absolutely impossible to script out every possible encounter that a student might have in the field, and thus it is impossible to anticipate all the ethical dilemmas that students may face. The best we can do is talk in a useful, constructive way about ethical issues and try to prevent students from taking unnecessary risks. I think a risk–benefit assessment is a worthwhile exercise, where the benefits that may be derived are weighed against the probable costs of obtaining such information. But ethics are always a matter of judgment, and judgments are always in flux.
>
> (Wolcott, 2010: 124)

As we have tried to illustrate in this chapter, ethics in qualitative research is a complex and dynamic process rather than a static product. No one researcher can solve all the dilemmas we have signalled but they do need to be aware of them and be able to adopt an informed and principled position if they are to engage with lives of people in SEH in a meaningful, respectful, fair and responsible manner.

CHAPTER 9

BRIEF REFLECTIONS

Originally, we conceptualised this book as evolving around the notion of qualitative research being both a dynamic process and a product that is cyclical in nature. The chapters as we have framed them were designed to take the reader on a journey though the process of conducting qualitative research starting with the initial conceptualising of ideas and questions, through the stages of data collection and analysis, and then onto how the findings of studies can be communicated to audiences in various ways. As part of this journey, we also considered how the quality of qualitative research might be judged, and reflected on the ethical issues that are inherent in this form of inquiry. Throughout the book, although there may be times when it is appropriate to seek a pre-existing 'off-the-shelf' methodology that someone else has developed which can be adopted for ready-made use, we have emphasised that in terms of both process and product, qualitative researchers need to make critical, informed, principled and strategic decisions as their study develops. This is because without such decisions being made, 'methodolatry' would prevail, with all that this entails, and qualitative research would not be worthy of its name, nor would it be able to justify itself as an important and necessary form of scholarship for understanding the social worlds of SEH.

Looking back, however, we recognise that what we have produced is not only a book that, hopefully, helps readers to conduct qualitative research but also something that helps them to justify and defend it against those who would deny its worth and legitimacy as a form of inquiry. With regard to the latter, Wolcott (1995) spoke with his usual eloquence of the *art of (conceptual) self-defence.* At the most obvious level, this kind of defence is necessary for qualitative researchers to use when attempting to defend their work against certain kinds of quantitative researcher who seem to combine a blinding arrogance with a woeful ignorance not only about qualitative research in general but any form of inquiry (including some quantitative work) that does not fit within their narrowly defined methodological remit and limited boundary of understanding. Of course, the same can be said for the ways in which certain qualitative researchers who, with no less arrogance and ignorance, wrongly demean quantitative research and blame those who practise it for a whole host of problems in the world both real and imaginary.

In terms of the qualitative camp itself and the traditions and communities (or is it tribes?) that make it up, some advocates are not averse to demeaning different traditions in the process of creating the negative 'Other'. Finally, as we have indicated in various chapters of this book, even within qualitative traditions and communities, there can be tensions and disputes that require the art of (conceptual) self-defence to be mobilised. In this regard, as Wolcott (1995) notes, certain problems or key issues keep recurring, not only in the dialogue between quantitative and qualitative researchers but also among qualitative researchers as well.

> Fieldworkers need perspectives and coping strategies for dealing with them. They do not need definitive answers that resolve the issues for all times, for these are the debates that surround the inquiry process itself . . . My advice to beginning researchers is to be informed as to the substance of these debates rather than being drawn prematurely into them . . . There are myriad issues, ethical, methodological, and philosophical, about which you may be asked or challenged to take a stand. If you are you will be expected to have a thoughtful position, not expected to come up with 'the answer' . . . Do not get lured into believing that the entire rationale for qualitative approaches now rests on your shoulders alone, or that until you have satisfactorily resolved each of these methodological perplexities, you may not proceed with your own research.
>
> (Wolcott, 1995: 159–160)

In terms of issues such as objectivity, generalisability, reliability and validity, Wolcott (1995) would argue that we as qualitative researchers, both individually and collectively,

> need to be thoughtfully aware of them, to have both a sense of the underlying problems they point to and a working resolution for them. My call is for fieldworkers to be well coached in the

art of self-defence, intrigued with, rather than defensive about, epistemological issues.

(p. 176)

Qualitative researchers have no need to be defensive or apologetic about their work. For example, Lincoln (2010) argues that those working in this field, especially those within a critical and openly ideological tradition, have been a powerful force for expanding knowledge of social processes, especially oppressive social practices, which remained largely obscured or glossed until the past quarter century. For her, the efforts of qualitative researchers have been instrumental in exposing, 'the clandestine disfigurements and outrages of racism, sexism, homophobia, and class injuries as well as the relentless marketization of sexuality, youth, and beauty' (p. 4).

According to Lincoln (2010) qualitative researchers should be *proud* of the stunning array of work they have turned out. She suggests they have become, largely because of their methods, lenses and paradigmatic stance, 'rather awesome purveyors of some of the most profound insights into Western society ever assembled' (p. 4). For Lincoln, qualitative researchers have seen the ugly underbelly of this society and been unfaltering and remorseless in exposing their shortcomings as a society to themselves and the rest of the world. She concludes as follows, 'In the past 25 years, the interpretivist, ethnographic, and critical community has produced a virtual tsunami of important critical work' (p. 4). We now have:

- Deep studies of teaching, learning and teacher practices;
- Deep and publicly accessible studies of hidden and oppressive infrastructures in our public schools;
- Thoughtful, trenchant, meticulously documented and damning studies of the effects of racism, gender discrimination and classism – in society, in the public schools, in higher education;
- Penetrating studies of the beneficial effects of diversity; and
- We are beginning to see hybridity, not as exotic and ambiguous, but as the bellwether of globalism. (Lincoln, 2010: 4)

This said, as Denzin (2009) suggests, given that the contributions qualitative research can make to knowedge is not well understood by many, we need to become better at educating policy-makers and other audiences, 'showing them how qualitative research and our views of practical science, interpretation, and performance ethics can positively contribute to projects embodying restorative justice, equity, and better schooling' (p. 81). Accordingly, as part of his agenda to promote and develop qualitative research, Denzin (2010) speaks of *advocacy*. Here, the qualitative community needs to develop systematic contacts with political figures, the media, professional associations and with practitioners such as teachers and health professionals in the field. Advocacy with such groups would include: (1) showing how qualitative work addresses issues of social policy; (2) critiquing federally and nationally mandated ethical guidelines for human subject research; and (3) critiquing outdated positivist modes of science and research.

Denzin (2010) also calls for an *operational* agenda, the goals of which should include building productive relationships with professional associations, journals, policy makers and funders. Representatives from many different professional associations, such as the sociological, anthropological, psychological, educational, health associations, and so on, of any individual country, need to be brought together.

Qualitative researchers, in short, need to emphasise and make clear to different constituencies and stakeholders the *benefits* that their work has in a variety of domains that range from the local to the international. These include the following:

- Qualitative research can generate new theories, adapt, develop and refine existing theoretical frameworks, and challenge taken-for-granted theories.
- Qualitative research can improve healthcare practices, improve the quality of life, and support better health outcomes for different groups within the population including athletes.
- Qualitative research can inform intervention programmes, generate behaviour change, and develop applied practices.
- Qualitative research can influence policy development and implementation, improve public services, make a difference to how practitioners work, and have a pedagogical impact at the user level.
- Qualitative research can contribute to the creative economy and contribute to cultural enrichment.
- Qualitative research can extend the global/national knowledge base beyond the academy and contribute to civil society, social justice, and the empowerment of individuals and groups.

In making clear the benefits of qualitative research and influencing the views of others about our work, Denzin (2009, 2010) argues that we need to find new strategic and tactical ways to work with one another in the new paradigm dialogue (see also Sparkes, 2013). This means that dialogues need to be formed between advocates of quantitative and qualitative research and between the various traditions that are contained within them.

> There needs to be a greater openness to alternative paradigms critiques . . . There needs to be a decline in conflict between alternative paradigms proponents. Paths for fruitful dialogue between and across paradigms need to be explored. This means that there needs to be a greater openness to and celebration of the proliferation, intermingling, and confluence of paradigms and interpretive frameworks.
>
> (Denzin, 2010: 40)

One area which has great potential for such intermingling and dialogue is that of *transdisciplinary research* (TDR). This is an emergent approach conducted by investigators from different disciplines working jointly to create new conceptual, theoretical, methodological and translational innovations that integrate and move beyond discipline-specific approaches to address a common problem. It has several characteristics that distinguish it from multi-disciplinary and inter-disciplinary approaches.

Multi-disciplinary refers to research in which each specialist remains within their discipline and contributes using disciplinary concepts and methods. Inter-disciplinary contributions can be interpreted as the bringing together of disciplines which retain their own concepts and methods that are applied to a mutually agreed subject. Based on a systematic literature review, interviews and field tests with inter-disciplinary researchers, Aboelela *et al.* (2007) define interdisciplinary research as 'any study or group of studies undertaken by scholars from two or more distinct scientific disciplines' (p. 341).

In contrast, drawing on Carew and Wickson (2010), and Wickson, Carew and Russell (2006), the main characteristics that constitute TDR and which make it different from multi- and inter-disciplinary approaches are as follows.

■ *Transcending, collaborating and integrating*: TDR transcends the traditional boundaries of university-based research to include the collaborative participation of academic stakeholders. While multi- and interdisciplinary research also involves some degree of collaboration, TDR broadens what constitutes collaboration. It is about intentionally involving the experiences of those people affected by the research. This includes involving such user-group members or stakeholders in the definition of problems and the objectives of the study along with how resources are used to analyse findings and apply them. In this regard, TDR is a collaborative knowledge-generation process between researchers and stakeholders. Besides transcending the boundaries of disciplines it is also important for TDR to transcend other boundaries, such as affect/effect or fact/value; and epistemological divides. In addition, TDR seeks to integrate these potentially disparate knowledges with a view to creating knowledge that can be applied in a given problem context and has some prospect of producing desired change for those involved.

■ *Practical problems, problem orientation*: Society is facing problems manifest in the real world that are messy, complex, multi-dimensional and not easily confined by the boundaries of a single disciplinary framework. TDR therefore aims to make practical contributions to the resolution of pressing problems as they manifest in their various social and physical contexts. The problems in question are not theoretical or abstracted, but exist within multi-layered, and contested everyday contexts. They tend to be those that are perceived or nominated by stakeholders or society in general as pressing and urgently in need of resolution. Accordingly, TDR starts with a problem that is 'in the world and actual' rather than 'in a researcher's head and conceptual'. Unlike in much multi- and inter-disciplinary research, the intent in TDR is to provide a 'solution' to a problem identified by stakeholders. In this sense, transdisciplinary researchers are similar to participatory action researchers and those engaged in cultural praxis research. In TDR there is also, however, the explicit aim of fusing different disciplinary knowledges with the know-how of stakeholders as well as the adoption of an evolving methodology.

■ *Evolving methodology*: Multidisciplinary research involves disciplines studying research themes using their own methodological approaches and retaining disciplinary autonomy. Interdisciplinary research involves developing a shared methodological framework within which distinct epistemological approaches are used to study different themes of a research problem. In contrast, TDR is characterised by an interpenetration or integration of different disciplinary methodologies and, ideally, epistemologies. Interpenetration refers to the evolution of research methods and methodologies via a process of scholars using multiple research approaches to critique and deconstruct those in use in their current study. This process champions the development of methods specifically tailored to the selected problem and its unique context. In terms of paradigmatic incommensurability, interpenetration does not, however, mean that researchers necessarily aim to reconcile and integrate approaches to research and research outcomes that rest on fundamentally different epistemological bases. In seeking to integrate different knowledges and epistemologies, transdisciplinary researchers do not need to develop a single unified 'truth.' Rather they can aim to integrate the different knowledges by looking for correspondences, coherence, and what Wickson *et al.* (2006) call 'ridges' across the differences, generating knowledge by finding, identifying and communicating patterns across diverse disciplines and discourses. Thus, TDR rejects methodological reductionism and adopts a pluralistic methodology.

TDR is not easy to engage with and sustain because the 'transcendence' necessary requires the giving up of sovereignty over knowledge, the creation of new insights and knowledge by collaboration, and the capacity to consider the know-how of professionals and lay-people. This said, when accomplished in a supportive environment, TDR has enormous potential to foster the cross-fertilisation of ideas and knowledge from different contributors that, in turn, can lead to new theories, a synergy of new methods, and an expanded understanding of a particular topic or problem. All these are essential if our current understanding of the interrelations between the different sciences with the field of SEH is to be improved.

Of course, as we have made clear throughout this book, the notion of seeking 'transcendence' does not just apply to those engaged in TDR. Rather, a dose of this would be valuable for researchers of all kinds as a way of encouraging an informed, respectful and fruitful dialogue within and between research paradigms, camps, communities and traditions. For Denzin (2010), this kind of dialogue is not only a possibility, 'it is a requirement if a democratic community is to flourish in the academy and within the qualitative research community. Strong academic departments encourage paradigm diversity' (p. 42). Paradigm diversity does not mean that we will all agree with each other all the time or that the tensions between and within different research approaches will dissolve. Rather, as we have stressed throughout this book, such diversity and difference is a creative resource that should be celebrated and honoured by scholars who are willing to engage knowingly and respectfully with others who may not share their views as part of a wider commitment to making the world a better place to live in for *all* its inhabitants and not just the privileged few who have the power to shape it in their own image and for their own purposes. As part of this venture, qualitative research has an essential role to play. Those who practice this form of inquiry should take pride in the different kinds of knowledge, understanding and awareness they contribute to SEH and look forward to the dynamic and innovative offerings they, as qualitative researchers, will undoubtably make in the future.

REFERENCES

Aboelela, S., Larson, E., Bakken, S., Carrasquillo, O., Formicola, A., Glied, S., Hass, J., & Gebbie, K. (2007). Defining interdisciplinary research: Conclusions from a critical review of the literature. *Health Services Research*, 42: 329–346.

Abramson, C., & Modzelewski, D. (2011). Caged morality: Moral worlds, subculture, and stratification among middle-class cage-fighters. *Qualitative Sociology*, 34: 143–175.

Agee, J. (2009). Developing qualitative research questions: A reflective process. *International Journal of Qualitative Studies in Education*, 22: 431–447.

Allen-Collinson, J. (2005). Emotions, interaction and the injured sporting body. *International Review for the Sociology of Sport*, 40: 221–240.

Allen-Collinson, J. (2008). Running the routes together: Corunning and knowledge in action. *Journal of Contemporary Ethnography*, 37: 38–61.

Allen-Collinson, J. (2009). Sporting embodiment: Sports studies and the (continuing) promise of phenomenology. *Qualitative Research in Sport, Exercise and Health*, 1: 279–296.

Allen-Collinson, J. (2012). Autoethnography: Situating personal sporting narratives in socio-cultural contexts. In K. Young & M. Atkinson (Eds.). *Qualitative research on sport and physical culture* (pp. 191–212). Bingley, UK: Emerald Group Publishing Ltd.

Allen-Collinson, J., & Hockey, J. (2005). Autoethnography: Self indulgence or rigorous methodology. In M. McNamee (Ed.), *Philosophy and the sciences of exercise, health and sport: Critical perspectives on research methods* (pp. 187–202). London: Routledge.

Allen-Collinson, J., & Hockey, J. (2011). Feeling the way: Notes towards a haptic phenomenology of distance running and scuba diving. *International Review for the Sociology of Sport*, 46: 330–345.

American Psychological Association (2009). *Publication Manual of the American Psychological Association (6th edition)*. Washington, DC: American Psychological Association.

Anderson, E., & Kian, E. (2012). Examining media contestation of masculinity and head trauma in the National Football League. *Men and Masculinities*, 15: 152–173.

246

Angrosino, M. (2007). *Doing ethnographic observational research*. London: Sage.

Apostolis, N., & Giles, A. (2011). Portrayals of women golfers in the 2008 issues of Golf Digest. *Sociology of Sport Journal*, 28: 226–238.

Atkinson, M. (2009). Parkour, anarcho-environmentalism and poiesis. *Journal of Sport and Social Issues*, 33: 169–194.

Atkinson, M. (2010). Fell running in post-sport territories. *Qualitative Research in Sport, Exercise and Health*, 2: 109–132.

Atkinson, M. (2012). The empirical strikes back: Doing realist ethnography. In K. Young & M. Atkinson (Eds.), *Qualitative research on sport and physical culture* (pp. 23–50). Bingley, UK: Emerald Group Publishing Ltd.

Atkinson, R. (1998). *The life story interview*. London: Sage.

Atkinson, R. (2007). The life story interview as a bridge in narrative inquiry. In D. J. Clandidnin (Ed.), *Handbook of narrative inquiry* (pp. 224–245). Thousand Oaks, CA: Sage.

Avis, M. (2005). Is there an epistemology for qualitative research? In I. Holloway (Ed.), *Qualitative research in health care* (pp. 3–17). Milton Keynes: Open University Press.

Bagley, C. (2009). The ethnographer as impresario-joker in the (re)presentation of educational research as performance art: Towards a performance ethic. *Ethnography and Education*, 4: 283–300.

Bagley, C. & Castro-Salazar, R. (2012). Critical arts-based research in education: Performing undocumented historias. *British Educational Research Journal*, 38: 219–239.

Banks, S. (2008). Writing as theory: In defence of fiction. In J. Knowles & A. Cole (Eds.), *Handbook of the arts in qualitative research,* (pp. 155–164). London: Sage.

Barone, T. (2000). *Aesthetics, politics, and educational inquiry*. New York: Peter Lang.

Barone, T. (2008). Creative nonfiction and social research. In J. G. Knowles & A. Cole (Eds.), *Handbook of the arts in qualitative research* (pp. 105–116). London: Sage.

Barone, T., & Eisner, E. (2012). *Arts based research*. London: Sage.

Beneito-Montagut, R. (2011). Ethnography goes online: Towards a user-centred methodology to research interpersonal communication on the internet. *Qualitative Research*, 11: 716–735.

Bergson, H. (1961). *An introduction to metaphysics* (M. L. Andison, Trans). New York: Philosophical library. (Originally published 1903).

Bernstein, R. (1991). *The new constellation: The ethical-political horizons of modernity/postmodernity*. Cambridge, UK: Polity Press.

Berry, K., Kowalski, K., Ferguson, L., & McHugh, T. (2010). An empirical phenomenology of young adult women exercisers' body self-compassion. *Qualitative Research in Sport, Exercise and Health*, 2: 293–312.

Berry, T. (2011). Qualitative researchers as modern day Sophists? Reflections on the qualitative–quantitative divide. *Qualitative Research in Sport, Exercise and Health*, 3, 324–328.

Bidonde, M., Goodwin, D., & Drinkwater, D. (2009). Older women's experiences of a fitness program: The importance of social networks. *Journal of Applied Sport Psychology*, 21: 86–101.

Blee, K., & Currier, A. (2011). Ethics beyond the IRB: An introductory essay. *Qualitative Sociology*, 34: 401–413.

Blodgett, A., Schinke, R., Smith, B., Peltier, D., & Pheasant, C. (2011). In indigenous words: Exploring vignettes as a narrative strategy for presenting the research voices of Aboriginal community members. *Qualitative Inquiry*, *17*, 522–533.

Bluff, R. (2005). Grounded theory: The methodology. In I. Holloway (Ed.), *Qualitative research in health care* (pp. 147–167). Milton Keynes: Open University Press.

Bogardus, L. (2012). The Bolt Wars: A social worlds perspective on rock climbing and intragroup conflict. *Journal of Contemporary Ethnography*, 41: 283–308.

Bolin, A., & Granskog, J. (Eds.), (2003). *Athletic intruders: Ethnographic research on women, culture, and exercise.* Albany: SUNY Press.

Bondi, L. (2013). Research and therapy: Generating meaning and feeling gaps. *Qualitative Inquiry*, 19: 9–19.

Boyle, E., Millington, B., Vertinsky, P. (2006). Representing the female pugilist: Narratives of race, gender and disability in *Million Dollar Baby*. *Sociology of Sport Journal*, 23: 99–116.

Braun, V., & Clarke, V. (2006). Using thematic analysis in psychology. *Qualitative Research in Psychology*, 3: 77–101.

Breeze, R. (2011). Critical discourse analysis and its critics. *Pragmatics*, 21: 493–525.

Bresler, L. (2008). The music lesson. In J. Knowles & A. Cole (Eds.), *Handbook of the arts in qualitative research* (pp. 225–237). London: Sage.

Brewer, J., & Sparkes, A. (2011). Young people living with parental bereavement: Insights from an ethnographic study of a UK childhood bereavement service. *Social Science and Medicine*, 72: 283–290.

Bringer, J., Brackenridge, C., & Johnston, L. (2006). Swimming coaches' perceptions of sexual exploitation in sport: A preliminary model of role conflict and role ambiguity. *The Sport Psychologist*, 20: 465–479.

Bringer, J., Johnston, L., & Brackenridge, C. (2006). Using computer-assisted qualitative data analysis software to develop a grounded theory project. *Field Methods*, 18: 245–266.

Brocki, J., & Wearden, A. (2006). A critical evaluation of the use of interpretive phenomenological analysis (IPA) in health psychology. *Psychology and Health*, 21: 87–108.

Brown, D. (2002). Going digital and staying qualitative: Some alternative strategies for digitizing the qualitative research process. *Forum: Qualitative Social Research*, 3. Available online: http://www.qualitative-research.net/fqs/fqs-eng.htm.

Brown, D., Jennings, G., & Sparkes, A. (2010) 'It can be a religion if you want': Wing Chun Kung Fu as a secular religion. *Ethnography*, 11: 533–557.

Brown, G., Gilbourne, D., & Claydon, J. (2009). When a career ends: A short story. *Reflective Practice*, 10: 491–500.

Brymer, E., & Schweitzer, R. (2012). Extreme sports are good for your health: A

248

phenomenological understanding of fear and anxiety in extreme sport. *Journal of Health Psychology.* DOI: 10.1177/1359105312446770.

Buchanan, E., & Zimmer, M. (2012). Internet Research Ethics. *The Stanford encyclopedia of philosophy* (Winter 2012 edition). Available online: http://plato.stanford.edu/archives/win2012/entries/ethics-internet-research/.

Burke, S., & Sabiston, C. (2010). The meaning of the mountain: Exploring breast cancer survivors' lived experience of subjective well-being during a climb on Mt. Kilimanjaro. *Qualitative Research in Sport, Exercise and Health*, 2: 1–16.

Burke, S., & Sparkes, A. (2009). Cognitive dissonance and the role of self in high altitude mountaineering: An analysis of six published autobiographies. *Life Writing*, 6: 329–347.

Burke, S., Sparkes, A., & Allen-Collinson, J. (2008). High altitude climbers as ethnomethodologists making sense of cognitive dissonance: Ethnographic insights from an attempt to scale Mt. Everest. *The Sport Psychologist*, 22: 336–355.

Busanich, R., McGannon, K., & Schinke, R. (2012). Expanding understandings of the body, food and exercise relationship in distance runners: A narrative approach. *Psychology of Sport and Exercise*, 13: 582–590.

Buscher, M., Urry, J., & Witchger, K. (2011). *Mobile methods.* London: Routledge.

Butryn, T. (2011). Dancing with quantiods: A brief and benevolent commentary on the special issue of QRSEH. *Qualitative Research in Sport, Exercise and Health*, 3: 385–393.

Camiré, M., Trudel, P., & Forneris, T. (2009). High school athletes' perspectives on support, negotiation processes, and life skill development. *Qualitative Research in Sport, Exercise and Health*, 1: 72–88.

Cannella, G., & Lincoln, Y. (2011). Ethics, research regulations, and critical social science. In N. Denzin & Y. Lincoln (Eds.), *Handbook of qualitative research* (4th ed., pp. 81–90). Thousand Oaks, CA: Sage.

Carew, A., & Wickson, F. (2010). The TD Wheel: A heuristic to shape, support and evaluate transdisciplinary research. *Futures*, 42: 1146–1155.

Carless, D. (2008). Narrative, identity and recovery from serious mental illness: A life history of a runner. *Qualitative Research in Psychology*, 5: 233–248.

Carless, D. (2012a). Negotiating sexuality and masculinity in school sport: An autoethnography. *Sport, Education and Society*, 17: 607–626.

Carless, D. (2012b). Young men, sport and sexuality: A poetic exploration. In F. Dowling, H. Fitzgerald & A. Flintoff (Eds.), *Equity and difference in physical education, youth sport and health: A narrative approach* (pp. 67–71). London: Routledge.

Carless, D., & Douglas, K. (2008). Narrative, identity and mental health: How men with serious mental illness re-story their lives through sport and exercise. *Psychology of Sport and Exercise*, 9: 576–594.

Carless, D., & Douglas, K. (2009a). Opening doors: Poetic representation of the sport experiences of men with severe mental health difficulties. *Qualitative Inquiry*, 15: 1547–1551.

Carless, D., & Douglas, K. (2009b). Songwriting and the creation of knowledge. In B. Bartleet & C. Ellis (Eds.), *Musical autoethnography: Creative explorations of the self through music* (pp. 23–38). Queensland: Australian Academic Press.

Carless, D., & Douglas, K. (2010a). *Sport and physical activity for mental health.* Oxford: Wiley-Blackwell.

Carless, D., & Douglas, K. (2010b). Performance ethnography as an approach to health-related education. *Educational Action Research*, 18: 373–388.

Carless, D., & Douglas, K. (2011). What's in a song? How songs contribute to the communication of social science research. *British Journal of Guidance and Counselling*, 39: 439–454.

Carless, D., & Sparkes, A. (2008). The physical activity experiences of men with serious mental illness: Three short stories. *Psychology of Sport and Exercise*, 9: 191–210.

Carson, F., & Polman, R. (2008). ACL injury rehabilitation: A psychological case study of a professional rugby union player. *Journal of Clinical Sport Psychology*, 2: 71–90.

Caudwell, J. (2006) (Ed.), *Sport, sexualities and queer/theory.* London: Routledge.

Caudwell, J. (2011). Sport feminism(s): Narratives of linearity? *Journal of Sport and Social Issues*, 35: 111–125.

Caudwell, J. (2012). Theorising women's sport participation: Debating sport feminisms. *Psychology of Women Section Review*, 14: 4–8.

Caulley, D. (2008) Making qualitative research reports less boring: The techniques of writing creative nonfiction. *Qualitative Inquiry*, 14: 424–449.

Chamberlain, K. (2011). Commentary: Troubling methodology. *Health Psychology Review*, 5: 48–54.

Chang, H. (2008). *Autoethnography as method.* Walnut Creek, CA: Left Coast Press Inc.

Charmaz, K. (2004). Premises, principles, and practices in qualitative research: Revisiting the foundations. *Qualitative Health Research*, 14: 976–993.

Charmaz, K. (2005). Grounded theory in the 21st Century. In N. Denzin & Y. Lincoln (Eds.), *The Handbook of Qualitative Research* (3rd ed., pp. 507–535). London: Sage.

Charmaz, K. (2006). *Constructing grounded theory: A practical guide through qualitative analysis.* London: Sage.

Charmaz, K. (2008). Grounded theory. In J. Smith (Ed.), *Qualitative psychology: A practical guide to research methods* (2nd ed., pp. 81–110). New York: Guilford.

Chawansky, M. (2011). The recruit. *Qualitative Research in Sport, Exercise and Health*, 3: 1–8.

Chenail, R. (2010). Getting specific about qualitative research generalizability. *Journal of Ethnographic and Qualitative Research*, 5: 1–11.

Chenail, R., Cooper, R., & Desir, C. (2010). Strategically reviewing the research literature in qualitative research. *Journal of Ethnographic and Qualitative Research*, 4: 88–94.

Cherrington, J., & Watson, B. (2010). Shooting a diary, not just a hoop: Using video diaries to explore the embodied everyday contexts of a university basketball team. *Qualitative Research in Sport, Exercise and Health*, 2: 267–281.

Cho, J., & Trent, A. (2006). Validity in qualitative research revisited. *Qualitative Research*, 6: 319–340.

Cho, J., & Trent, A. (2009). Validity criteria for performance-related qualitative work: Towards a reflexive, evaluative and co-constructive framework for performance in/as qualitative inquiry. *Qualitative Inquiry*, 15: 1013–1041.

Christians, C. (2005). Ethics and politics in qualitative research. In N. Denzin & Y. Lincoln (Eds.), *Handbook of qualitative research* (3rd ed., pp. 139–164). Thousand Oaks, CA: Sage.

Clegg, J., & Butryn, T. (2012). An existential phenomenological examination of parkour and free running. *Qualitative Research in Sport, Exercise and Health*, 4: 320–340.

Coffey, A., & Atkinson, P. (1996). *Making sense of qualitative data: Complementary research strategies*. Thousand Oaks, CA: Sage.

Collingridge, D., & Gantt, E. (2008). The quality of qualitative research. *American Journal of Medical Quality*, 23: 389–395.

Corbin, J., & Strauss, A. (2007). *Basics of qualitative research: Techniques and procedures for developing grounded theory*. London: Sage.

Corden, A., & Sainsbury, R. (2006). Exploring 'quality': Research participants' perspectives on verbatim quotations. *International Journal of Social Research Methodology*, 9: 97–110.

Cosh, S., LeCouteur, A., Crabb, S., & Kettler, L. (2013). Career transitions and identity: A discursive psychological approach to exploring athlete identity in the transition back into elite sport. *Qualitative Research in Sport, Exercise and Health*, 5: 21–42.

Creswell, J. (2007). *Qualitative inquiry and research design: Choosing among five traditions*. London: Sage.

Crossley, M. (2000). *Introducing narrative psychology*. Buckingham, UK: Open University Press.

Crust, L., Keegan, R., Piggott, D., & Swann, C. (2011). Walking the walk: A phenomenological study of long distance walking. *Journal of Applied Sport Psychology*, 23: 243–262.

Culver, D., Gilbert, W., & Sparkes, A. (2012). Qualitative research in sport psychology journals: The next decade 2000–2009 and beyond. *The Sport Psychologist*, 26: 261–281.

D'Abundo, M. (2009). Issues of health, appearance and physical activity in aerobic classes for women. *Sport, Education and Society*, 14: 301–320.

D'Alonzo, K., & Sharma, M. (2010). The influence of *marianismo* beliefs on physical activity of mid-life immigrant latinas: A photovoice study. *Qualitative Research in Sport, Exercise and Health*, 2: 229–249.

Damianakis, T., & Woodford, M. (2012). Qualitative research with small connected communities: Generating new knowledge while upholding research ethics. *Qualitative Health Research*, 22: 708–718.

Dart, J. (2012). Sports review: A content analysis of the *International Review for the Sociology of Sport*, the *Journal of Sport and Social Issues* and the *Sociology of Sport Journal* across 25 years. *International Review for the Sociology of Sport*. DOI: 10.1177/1012690212465736.

Davis, N., & Meyer, B. (2009). Qualitative data analysis: A procedural comparison. *Journal of Applied Sport Psychology*, 21: 116–124.

Day, M., Bond, K., & Smith, B. (2013). Holding it together: Coping with vicarious trauma in sport. *Psychology of Sport and Exercise*, 14: 1–11.

Day, M., & Thatcher, J. (2009). 'I'm really embarrassed that you're going to read this . . .': Reflections on using diaries in qualitative research. *Qualitative Research in Psychology*, 6: 249–259.

Day, S. (2012). A reflexive lens: Exploring dilemmas of qualitative methodology through the concept of reflexivity. *Qualitative Sociology Review*, 8: 60–85.

Delmar, C. (2010). 'Generalizability' as recognition: Reflections on a foundational problem in qualitative research. *Qualitative Studies*, 1: 115–128.

Denison, J., & Markula, P. (Eds.), (2003). *Moving writing: Crafting movement in sport research*. New York: Peter Lang.

Denzin, N. (1997). *Interpretive ethnography: Ethnographic practices for the 21st century*. London: Sage.

Denzin, N. (2009). *Qualitative inquiry under fire*. Walnut Creek, CA: Left Coast press.

Denzin, N. (2010). *The qualitative manifesto: A call to arms*. Walnut Creek, CA: Left Coast Press.

Denzin, N., & Lincoln, Y. (1994). Introduction: Entering the field of qualitative research. In N. Denzin & Y. Lincoln (Eds.), *Handbook of qualitative research* (pp. 1–17). London: Sage.

Denzin, N., & Lincoln, Y. (2000). Introduction: The discipline and practice of qualitative research. In N. Denzin & Y. Lincoln (Eds.), *Handbook of qualitative research* (2nd ed., pp. 1–29). London: Sage.

Denzin, N., & Lincoln, Y. (2005). Introduction: The discipline and practice of qualitative research. In N. Denzin & Y. Lincoln (Eds). *The Sage handbook of qualitative research* (3rd ed., ix–xix). London: Sage.

Dickson-Swift, V., James, E., Kippen, S., & Liamputtong, P. (2007). Doing sensitive research: What challenges do qualitative researchers face? *Qualitative Research*, 7: 327–353.

Dingwell, R. (1992). 'Don't mind him – he's from Barcelona': Qualitative methods in health studies. In J. Daly, I. McDonald & E. Willis (Eds.), *Researching health care: Designs, dilemmas and disciplines* (pp. 161–175). London: Routledge.

Douglas, K. (2009). Storying myself: Negotiating a relational identity in professional sport. *Qualitative Research in Sport, Exercise and Health*, 1: 176–190.

Douglas, K. (2012). Signals and signs. *Qualitative Inquiry*, 18: 525–532.

Douglas, K. & Carless, D. (2008). Nurturing a performative self. *Forum Qualitative Sozialforschung / Forum: Qualitative Social Research*, 9: Art. 23, http://www.qualitative-research.net/fqs-texte/2-08/08-2-23-e.htm.

Douglas, K., & Carless, D. (2009). Exploring taboo issues in professional sport though a fictional approach. *Reflective Practice*, 10: 311–323.

Douglas, K., & Carless, D. (2010). Restoring connections in physical activity and mental health research and practice: A confessional tale. *Qualitative Research in Sport, Exercise and Health*, 2: 336–353.

Dowling, F., & Flintoff, A. (2011). Getting beyond normative interview talk of sameness and celebrating difference. *Qualitative Research in Sport, Exercise and Health*, 3: 63–79.

Drummond, M. (2010). The natural: An autoethnography of a masculinized body in sport. *Men and Masculinities*, 12: 373–389.

Dunn, J., & Holt, N. (2004). A qualitative investigation of a personal-disclosure mutual-sharing team building activity. *The Sport Psychologist*, 18: 363–380.

Dupuis, S., Whyte, C., Carson, J., Genoe, L., Meshino, L., & Sadler, L. (2012). Just dance with me: An authentic partnership approach to understanding leisure in the dementia context. *World Leisure Journal*, 54: 240–254.

Dzikus, L., Fisher, L., & Hays, K. (2012). Shared responsibility: A case of and for 'real life' ethical decision-making in sport psychology. *The Sport Psychologist*, 26: 519–539.

Edwards, R., & Mauthner, M. (2012). Ethics and feminist research: Theory and practice. In T. Miller, M. Birch, M. Mauthner & J. Jessop (Eds.), *Ethics in qualitative research* (2nd ed., pp.14–28). London: Sage.

Eisner, E. (1991). *The enlightened eye: Qualitative inquiry and the enhancement of educational practice.* New York: Macmillan.

Eisner, E. (2008). Art and knowledge. In J. Knowles & A. Cole (Eds.), *Handbook of the arts in qualitative research* (pp. 3–12). London: Sage.

Eklund, R., Jeffery, K., Dobersek, U., & Cho, S. (2011). Reflections on qualitative research in sport psychology. *Qualitative Research in Sport, Exercise and Health*, 3: 285–290.

Ellis, C. (2007). Telling secrets, revealing lies: Relational ethics in intimate research with others. *Qualitative Inquiry*, 13: 3–29.

Ellis, C., & Bochner, A. (2000) Autoethnography, personal narrative, reflexivity: Researcher as subject. In N. Denzin & Y. Lincoln (Eds.), *Handbook of qualitative research* (2nd ed., pp. 733–768). London: Sage.

Etherington, K. (2004). *Becoming a reflexive researcher.* London: Jessica Kingsley Publisher.

Fairclough, N. (2010). *Critical discourse analysis: The critical study of language* (2nd ed.). Harlow: Longman.

Finlay, L., & Gough, B. (2003). *Reflexivity: A practical guide for researchers in health and the social sciences.* Oxford: Blackwell.

Finley, N. (2010). Skating femininity: Gender manoeuvring in woman's roller derby. *Journal of Contemporary Ethnography*, 39: 359–387.

Fitzpatrick, K. (2012). 'That's how the light gets in': Poetry, self and representation in ethnographic research. *Cultural Studies–Critical Methodologies*, 12: 8–14.

Flyvbjerg, B. (2001). *Making social science matter: Why social inquiry fails and how it can succeed again.* Cambridge: Cambridge University Press.

Flyvbjerg, B. (2006). Five misunderstandings about case-study research. *Qualitative Inquiry*, 12: 219–245.

Fortune, D., & Mair, H. (2011). Notes from the sports club: Confessional tales of two researchers. *Journal of Contemporary Ethnography*, 40: 457–484.

Frank, A. (1995). *The wounded storyteller: Body, illness, and ethics.* Chicago, IL: University of Chicago Press.

Frank, A. (2012). Practicing dialogical narrative analysis. In J. Holstein & J. Gubrium (Eds.), *Varieties of narrative analysis* (pp. 33–52). Los Angeles, CA: Sage.

Franklin, P., Rowland, E., Fox, R., & Nicolson, P. (2012). Research ethics in accessing hospital staff and securing informed consent. *Qualitative Health Research*, 22: 1727–1738.

Freeman, M. (2011). Validity in dialogic encounters with hermeneutic truths. *Qualitative Inquiry*, 17: 543–551.

Fusco, C. (2012). Critical feminist/queer methodologies: Deconstructing (hetero)normative inscriptions. In K. Young & M. Atkinson (Eds.). *Qualitative research on sport and physical culture* (pp. 151–166). Bingley, UK: Emerald Group Publishing Ltd.

Galli, N. & Vealey, R. (2008). 'Bouncing back' from adversity: Athletes' experiences of resilience. *The Sport Psychologist*, 22: 316–335.

Gaskin, C., Andersen, M., & Morris, T. (2010). Sport and physical activity in the life of a man with cerebral palsy: Compensation for disability with psychosocial benefits and costs. *Psychology of Sport and Exercise,* 11: 197–205.

Gibson, K. (2012a). Knight's children: Techno-science, consumerism and running shoes. *Qualitative Research in Sport, Exercise and Health*, 4: 341–361.

Gibson, K. (2012b). Two (or more) feet are better than one: Mixed methods research in sport and physical culture. In K. Young & M. Atkinson (Eds.). *Qualitative research on sport and physical culture* (pp. 213–232). Bingley, UK: Emerald Group Publishing Ltd.

Giges, B., & Van Raalte, J. (2012). Special issue of *The Sport Psychologist* case studies in sport psychology introduction. *The Sport Psychologist*, 26: 483–484.

Gilbourne, D. (2002). Sports participation, sports injury and images of self: An autobiographical narrative of a life-long legacy. *Reflective Practice*, 3: 71–78.

Gilbourne, D. (2010). 'Edge of Darkness' and 'Just in Time': Two cautionary tales, two styles, one story. *Qualitative Inquiry*, 16: 325–331.

Gilbourne, D. (2011). Just-in-time: A reflective poetic monologue. *Reflective Practice: International and Interdisciplinary Perspectives*, 12: 27–33.

Gill, D. (2011). Beyond the qualitative–quantitative dichotomy: Notes from a non-qualitative researcher. *Qualitative Research in Sport, Exercise and Health*, 3: 305–312.

Giorgi, A. (1985). *Phenomenology and psychological research*. Pittsburgh, PA: Duquesne University Press.

Giorgi, A. (2011). IPA and science: A response to Jonathan Smith. *Journal of Phenomenological Psychology*, 42: 195–216.

Glaser, B. (1978). *Theoretical sensitivity: Advances in the methodology of grounded theory*. Mill Valley, CA: The Sociology Press.

Glaser, B., & Strauss, A. (1967). *The discovery of grounded theory*. London: Sage.

Glesne, G., & Peshkin, A. (1992). *Becoming qualitative researchers: An introduction*. London: Longman Group Ltd.

Gold, R. (1958). Roles in sociological field observation. *Social Forces*, 36: 217–223.

Goldblatt, H., Karnieli-Miller, O., & Neumann, M. (2011). Sharing qualitative research findings with participants: Study experiences of methodological and ethical dilemmas. *Patient Education and Counselling*, *82* (3), 205–214.

Gravestock, H. (2010). Embodying understanding: Drawing as research in sport and exercise. *Qualitative Research in Sport, Exercise and Health*, 2: 196–208.

Gray, R., & Sinding, C. (2002). *Standing ovation*. Walnut Creek, CA: Altamira Press.

Green, J., & Thorogood, N. (2009). *Qualitative methods for health research* (2nd ed.). London: Sage.

Griffin, M. (2010). Setting the scene: Hailing women into a running identity. *Qualitative Research in Sport, Exercise and Health*, 2: 153–174.

Griffin, M. (2012). Health consciousness, running and female bodies: An ethnographic study of 'Active Ageing'. Exeter University, unpublished doctoral thesis.

Griggs, G. (2011). Ethnographic study of alternative sports by alternative means: List mining as a method of data collection. *Journal of Empirical Research on Human Research Ethics*, 6: 85–91.

Groom, R., Cushion, C., & Nelson, L. (2011). The delivery of video-based performance analysis by england youth soccer coaches: Towards a grounded theory. *Journal of Applied Sport Psychology*, 23: 16–32.

Guba, E., & Lincoln, Y. (1989). *Fourth generation evaluation*. London: Sage.

Guba, E., & Lincoln, Y. (1994). Competing paradigms in qualitative research. In N. Denzin & Y. Lincoln (Eds.), *Handbook of qualitative research* (pp. 105–117). London: Sage. .

Guba, E., & Lincoln, Y. (2005). Paradigmatic controversies, contradictions, and emerging confluences. In N. Denzin & Y. Lincoln (Eds.), *Handbook of qualitative research* (3rd ed., pp. 191–216). London: Sage.

Gubrium, J., & Holstein, J. (1997). *The new language of qualitative method*. Oxford: Oxford University Press.

Gubrium, J., & Holstein, J. (1998). Narrative practice and the coherence of personal stories. *Sociological Quarterly*, 39: 163–187.

Gubrium, J., & Holstein, J. (2002). *Handbook of interview research*. Thousand Oaks, CA: Sage.

Gubrium, J., & Holstein, J. (2008). The constructionist mosaic. In J. Holstein & J. Gubrium (Eds.), *Handbook of constructionist research* (pp. 3–10). London: The Guilford Press.

Gubrium, J., & Holstein, J. (2009). *Analyzing narrative reality*. London: Sage.

Hagger, M., & Chatzisarantis, N. (2011). Never the twain shall meet? Quantitative psychological researchers' perspectives on qualitative research. *Qualitative Research in Sport, Exercise and Health*, 3: 266–277.

Halkier, B. (2011). Methodological practicalities in analytical generalization. *Qualitative Inquiry*, 17: 787–797.

Hall, G., Shearer, D., Thomson, R., Roderique-Davies, G., Mayer, P., & Hall, R. (2012). Conceptualising commitment: A thematic analysis of fans of Welsh rugby. *Qualitative Research in Sport, Exercise and Health*, 4: 138–153.

Hammell, K. (2007). Quality of life after spinal cord injury: A meta-synthesis of qualitative findings. *Spinal Cord*, 45: 124–139.

Hammersley, M. (2009). Against the ethicists: On the evils of ethical regulation. *International Journal of Social Research Methodology*, 12: 211–225.

Hanna, P. (2012). Using internet technologies (such as Skype) as a research medium: A research note. *Qualitative Research*, 12: 239–242.

Hanold, M. (2010). Beyond the marathon: (De)constructing of female ultrarunning bodies. *Sociology of Sport Journal*, 27: 160–177.

Hare, R., Evans, L, & Callow, N. (2008). Imagery use during rehabilitation from injury: A case study of an elite athlete. *The Sport Psychologist*, 22: 405–422.

Hargreaves, J., & Vertinsky, P. (2007) (Eds.), *Physical culture, power, and the body*. London: Routledge.

Harper, D. (2005). What's new visually? In N. Denzin & Y. Lincoln (Eds.), *Handbook of qualitative research* (3rd ed., pp. 747–762). Thousand Oaks, CA: Sage.

Hart, N., & Crawford-Wright, A. (1999). Research as therapy, therapy as research: Ethical dilemmas in new-paradigm research. *British Journal of Guidance and Counselling*, 27: 205–214.

Harvey, J., Wilkinson, S., Pressé, C., Joober, R., & Grizenko, N. (2012). Scrapbook interviewing and children with attention-deficit hyperactivity disorder. *Qualitative Research in Sport, Exercise and Health*, 4: 62–79.

Harwood, C., Drew, A., & Knight, C. (2010). Parental stressors in professional youth football academies: A qualitative investigation of specialising stage parents. *Qualitative Research in Sport, Exercise and Health*, 2: 39–55.

Hatch, J., & Wisniewski, R. (Eds.). (1995). *Life history and narrative*. Lewes: Falmer Press.

Haverkamp, B., & Young, R. (2007). Paradigms, purpose, and the role of the literature formulating a rationale for qualitative investigations. *The Counselling Psychologist*, 35: 265–294.

Heil, J. (2012). Pain on the run: Injury, pain and performance in a distance runner. *The Sport Psychologist*, 26: 540–550.

Herzog, T., & Hays, K. (2012). Therapist or mental skills coach? How to decide. *The Sport Psychologist*, 26: 486–499.

Hewitt, J. (2007). Ethical components of researcher-researched relationships in qualitative interviewing. *Qualitative Health Research*, 17: 1149–1159.

Hockey, J. (2006). Sensing the run: The senses and distance running. *Senses and Society*, 1: 183–202.

Hockey, J. (2013). Knowing the 'Going': The sensory evaluation of distance running. *Qualitative Research in Sport, Exercise and Health*, 5: 127–141.

Hockey, J., & Allen-Collinson, J. (2007). Grasping the phenomenology of sporting bodies. *International Review for the Sociology of Sport*, 42: 115–131.

Holloway, I. (1997). *Basic concepts for qualitative research*. Oxford: Blackwell Science.

Holman Jones, S. (2005). Autoethnography: Making the personal political. In N. Denzin & Y. Lincoln (Eds.), *Handbook of qualitative research* (3rd ed., pp. 763–792). London: Sage.

Holt, N. & Sparkes, A. (2001). An ethnographic study of cohesiveness in a college soccer team over a season. *The Sport Psychologist*, 15: 237–259.

Holt, N., & Tamminen, K. (2010a). Improving grounded theory research in sport and exercise psychology: A response to Mike Weed. *Psychology of Sport and Exercise*, 11: 405–413.

Holt, N., & Tamminen, K. (2010b). Moving forward with grounded theory research in sport and exercise psychology. *Psychology of Sport and Exercise*, 11: 419–422.

Holt, N., Tamminen, K., Black, D., Sehn, Z., & Wall, M. (2008). Parental involvement in competitive youth sport settings. *Psychology of Sport and Exercise*, 9: 663–685.

256

Holt, N., Tamminen, K., Tink, L., & Black, D. (2009). An interpretive analysis of life skills associated with sport participation. *Qualitative Research in Sport, Exercise and Health*, 1: 160–175.

Hookway, N. (2008). 'Entering the blogosphere': Some strategies for using blogs in social research. *Qualitative Research*, 8: 91–113.

Horn, T. (2011). Multiple pathways to knowledge generation: Qualitative and quantitative research approaches in sport and exercise psychology. *Qualitative Research in Sport, Exercise and Health*, 3: 291–304.

Howells, K., & Grogan, S. (2012). Body image and the female swimmer: Muscularity but in moderation. *Qualitative Research in Sport, Exercise and Health*, 4: 98–116.

Hsieh, H., & Shannon, S. (2005). Three approaches to qualitative content analysis. *Qualitative Health Research*, 15: 1277–1288.

Hutchinson, A, Johnston, L., Breckon, J. (2011). Grounded theory-based research within exercise psychology: A critical review. *Qualitative Research in Psychology*, 8: 247–272.

Hutchinson, A, Johnston, L., Breckon, J. (2013). A grounded theory of successful long-term physical activity behavior change. *Qualitative Research in Sport, Exercise and Health*, 5: 109–126.

Johnson, B., & Russell, K. (2012). The construction of gendered bodies within competitive swimming: A Foucauldian perspective. *Psychology of Women Section Review*, 14: 26–33.

Johnson, M., Tenenbaum, G., Edmonds, W., & Castillo, Y. (2008). A comparison of the developmental experiences of elite and sub-elite swimmers: similar developmental histories can lead to differences in performance level. *Sport, Education and Society*, 13(4), 453–475.

Jones, M., & Lavallee, D. (2009). Exploring perceived life skills development and participation in sport. *Qualitative Research in Sport, Exercise and Health*, 1: 36–50.

Jones, R. (2006). Dilemmas, Maintaining 'face' and paranoia: An average coaching life. *Qualitative Inquiry*, 12: 1012–1021.

Jorgensen, D. (1989). *Participant observation*. London: Sage.

Kaiser, K. (2009). Protecting respondent confidentiality in qualitative research. *Qualitative Health Research*, 19: 1632–1641.

Kauer, K., & Krane, V. (2012). Heteronormative landscapes: Exploring sexuality through elite women athletes. *Psychology of Women Section Review*, 14: 10–17.

Kavanagh, E. (2012). Affirmation through disability: One athlete's personal journey to the London Paralympic Games. *Perspectives in Public Health*, 32: 68–74.

Kelly, J. (2010). 'Sectarianism' and Scottish football: Critical reflections on dominant discourse and press commentary. *International Review for the Sociology of Sport*, 46: 418–435.

Kerr, A., & Emery, P. (2011). Foreign fandom and the Liverpool FC: A cyber-mediated romance. *Soccer and Society*, 12: 880–896.

Kerr, J. (2007). Sudden withdrawal from skydiving: A case study informed by reversal theory's concept of protective frames. *Journal of Applied Sport Psychology*, 19: 337–351.

Kerr, J., & Males, J. (2010). The experience of losing: A qualitative study of elite lacrosse athletes and team performance at a world championship. *Psychology of Sport and Exercise*, 11: 394–401.

Kerry, D., & Amour, K. (2000). Sports science and the promise of phenomenology: philosophy, methods, and insight. *Quest*, 52: 1–17.

Kerry-Moran, K. (2008). Between scholarship and art: dramaturgy and quality in arts-related research. In J. Knowles & A. Cole (Eds.), *Handbook of the arts in qualitative research* (pp. 493–502). London: Sage.

Kluge, M., Grant, B., Friend, L., & Glick, L. (2010). Seeing is believing: Telling the 'inside' story of a beginning masters athlete through film. *Qualitative Research in Sport, Exercise and Health*, 2: 282–292.

Knight, C., Neely, K., & Holt, N. (2011). Parental behavior in team sports: How do female athletes want parents to behave? *Journal of Applied Sport Psychology*, 23: 76–92.

Knowles, J., & Cole, A. (2008). Preface. In J. Knowles & A. Cole (Eds.), *Handbook of the arts in qualitative research* (pp. xi–xiv). London: Sage.

Knowles, J., & Cole, A. (Eds.) (2008). *Handbook of the arts in qualitative research*. London: Sage.

Koro-Ljungberg, M. (2010). Validity and validation in the making in the context of qualitative research. *Qualitative Health Research*, 18: 983–989.

Krane, V. (2009). A sport odyssey. *Qualitative Research in Sport, Exercise and Health*, 1: 221–238.

Krane, V., & Baird, S. (2005). Using ethnography in applied sport psychology. *Journal of Applied Sport Psychology*, 17: 87–107.

Krane, V., Ross, S., Miller, M., Rowse, J., Ganoe, K., Andrzejczyk, J., & Lucas, C. (2010). Power and focus: Self-representation of female college athletes. *Qualitative Research in Sport, Exercise and Health*, 2: 175–195.

Krane, V., Walson, J., Kauer, K., & Semerjian, T. (2010). Queering sport psychology, in Ryba, T., Schinke, R., & Tenenbaum, G. (Eds.). *The cultural turn in sport psychology* (pp.153–180). Morgantown, WV: Fitness Information Technology.

Kvale, S., & Brinkmann, S. (2009). *Interviews: Learning the craft of qualitative research interviewing*. Thousand Oaks, CA: Sage.

Lafrance, M. (2011). Reproducing, resisting and transcending discourses of femininity: A discourse analysis of women's accounts of leisure'. *Qualitative Research in Sport, Exercise and Health*, 3: 80–98.

Lahman, M., Geist, M., Rodriguez, K., Graglia, P., & DeRoche, K. (2011). Culturally responsive relational reflexive ethics in research: The three Rs. *Quality and Quantity*, 45: 1397–1414.

Lang, M. (2010). Surveillance and conformity in competitive youth swimming'. *Sport, Education and Society*, 15: 19–37.

Lieblich, A., Tuval-Mashiach, R., & Zilber, T. (1998). *Narrative research: Reading, analysis and interpretation*. Thousand Oaks, CA: Sage.

Lincoln, Y. (2010). 'What a long, strange trip it's been': Twenty-five years of qualitative and new paradigm research. *Qualitative Inquiry*, 16: 3–9.

Lincoln, Y. & Guba, E. (1985). *Naturalistic inquiry*. Thousand Oaks, CA: Sage.

Lugosi, P. (2006). Between overt and covert research: Concealment and disclosure in an ethnographic study of commercial hospitality. *Qualitative Inquiry*, 12: 541–561.

Lundkvist, E. Gustafsson, H., Hjälm, S., & Hassmén, P. (2012). An interpretative phenomenological analysis of burnout and recovery in elite soccer coaches. *Qualitative Research in Sport, Exercise and Health*, 4: 400–419.

Mackenzie, S., & Kerr, J. (2012). Head-mounted cameras and stimulated recall in qualitative sport research. *Qualitative Research in Sport, Exercise and Health*, 4: 51–61.

Madill, A., & Gough, B. (2009). Qualitative research and its place in psychological science. *Psychological Methods*, 13: 254–271.

Markham, A. (2004). Internet communication as a tool for qualitative research. In D. Silverman (Ed.), *Qualitative research: Theory, method, and practices* (2nd ed., pp. 328–344). London: Sage.

Markham, A., & Buchanan, E. (2012). Ethical decision-making and internet research: Version 2.0: Recommendations from the AoIR Ethics Working Committee. Available online: *aoir.org/reports/ethics2.pdf*.

Markula, P., & Pringle R. (2006). *Foucault, sport and exercise: Power, knowledge and transforming the self*. London: Routledge.

Martin, J. (2011). Qualitative research in sport and exercise psychology: Observations of a non-qualitative researcher. *Qualitative Research in Sport, Exercise and Health*, 3: 335–348.

Martos-Garcia, D., Devis-Devis, J. & Sparkes, A. (2009). Sport and physical activity in a high security Spanish prison: An ethnographic study of multiple meanings. *Sport, Education and Society*, 14: 57–76.

Massey, W., Meyer, B., & Naylor, A. (2013). Toward a grounded theory of self-regulation in mixed martial arts. *Psychology of Sport and Exercise*, 14: 12–20.

Mauthner, M., Birch, M., Miller, T., & Jessop, J. (2012). Conclusion: Navigating ethical dilemmas and new digital horizons. In T. Miller, M. Birch, M. Mauthner & J. Jessop (Eds.), *Ethics in qualitative research* (2nd ed., pp. 176–186). London: Sage.

Maxwell, J. (1996). *Qualitative research design*. London: Sage.

Maykut, P., & Morehouse, R. (1994). *Beginning qualitative research: A philosophic and practical guide*. London: The Falmer Press.

McCarthy, P., & Jones, M. (2007). A qualitative study of sport enjoyment in the sampling years. *The Sport Psychologist*, 21: 400–416.

McDonough, M., Sabiston, C., & Crocker, P. (2008). An interpretive phenomenological examination of psychological changes among breast cancer survivors in their first season of Dragon Boat racing. *Journal of Applied Sport Psychology*, 20: 445–450.

McGannon, K. & Busanich, R. (2010). Rethinking subjectivity in sport and exercise psychology: A feminist post-structuralist perspective on women's embodied physical activity. In T. Ryba, R. Schinke & G. Tenenbaum (Eds.), *The cultural turn in sport psychology* (pp. 203–229). Morgantown, WV: Fitness Information Technology. doi: 10.1177/0193723501252004.

McGannon, K., Hoffmann, M., Metz, J., & Schinke, R. (2011). A media analysis of a sport celebrity: Understanding an informal 'team cancer' role as a socio-cultural construction. *Psychology of Sport and Exercise*, 13: 26–35.

McGannon, K., & Spence, J. (2010). Speaking of the self and understanding physical activity participation: What discursive psychology can tell us about an old problem. *Qualitative Research in Sport, Exercise and Health*, 2: 17–38.

McGannon, K., & Spence, J. (2012). Exploring news media representations of women's exercise and subjectivity through critical discourse analysis. *Qualitative Research in Sport, Exercise and Health*, 4: 32–50.

McGrath, S., & Chananie-Hill, R. (2009). 'Big freaky-looking women': Normalizing gender transgression through bodybuilding. *Sociology of Sport Journal*, 26: 235–254.

McKay, J., & Roderick, M. (2010). 'Lay down Sally': Media narratives of failure in Australian sport. *Journal of Australian Studies*, 34: 295–315.

McKee, H. A., & Porter, J. E. (2009). *The ethics of internet research: A rhetorical, case-based process*. New York: Peter Lang.

McKenna J., & Thomas H. (2007). Enduring injustice: A case study of retirement from professional rugby union. *Sport, Education and Society*, 12: 19–35.

McMahon, J., & Dinan-Thompson, M. (2011). Body work – Regulation of a swimmer body: An autoethnography from an Australian elite swimmer. *Sport, Education and Society*, 16: 35–50.

McMahon, J., Penney, D., & Dinan-Thompson, M. (2012). Body practices – exposure and effect of sporting culture? Stories from three Australian swimmers. *Sport, Education and Society*, 17: 181–206.

McMaster, S., Culver, D., & Werthner, P. (2012). Coaches of athletes with physical disability: A look at their learning experiences. *Qualitative Research in Sport, Exercise and Health*, 4: 226–243.

Medved, M., & Brockmeier, J. (2004). Making sense of traumatic experiences: Telling a life with fragile X syndrome. *Qualitative Health Research*, 14: 741–759.

Mellick, M., & Fleming, S. (2010). Personal narrative and the ethics of disclosure: A case study from elite sport. *Qualitative Research*, 10: 299–314.

Mienczakowski, J., & Moore, T. (2008). Performing data with notions of responsibility. In J. Knowles & A. Cole (Eds.), *Handbook of the arts in qualitative research* (pp. 451–458). London: Sage.

Millington, B., & Wilson, B. (2012). Media analysis in physical cultural studies: From production to reception. In K. Young & M. Atkinson (Eds.), *Qualitative research on sport and physical culture* (pp. 129–150). Bingley, UK: Emerald Group Publishing Ltd.

Millward, P. (2008). The rebirth of the football fanzine: Using e-zines as data source. *Journal of Sport and Social Issues*, 32: 299–310.

Monaghan, L. (2001). *Bodybuilding, drugs and risk*. London: Routledge.

Morse, J. (1999). Qualitative generalizability. *Qualitative Health Research*, 9: 5–6.

Morse, J. (2007). Ethics in action: Ethical principles for doing qualitative health research. *Qualitative Health Research*, 17: 1003–1005

Nicholls, A., Holt, N., & Polman, R. (2005). A phenomenological analysis of coping effectiveness in golf. *Sport Psychologist*, 19, 111–130.

Norlyk, A., & Harder, I. (2010). What makes a phenomenological study phenomenological? An analysis of peer-reviewed empirical nursing studies. *Qualitative Health Research*, 20: 420–431.

260

O'Reilly, K. (2012). *Ethnographic methods* (2nd ed.) London: Routledge.

Olive, R., & Thorpe, H. (2011). Negotiating the 'f-word' in the field: Doing feminist ethnography in action sport cultures. *Sociology of Sport Journal*, 28: 421–440.

Overman, S. (2008). *Living out of bounds: The male athlete's everyday life*. Westport, CT: Praeger Publishers.

Palmer, C., & Thompson, K. (2010). Everyday risks and professional dilemmas: Field work with alcohol-based (sporting) subcultures. *Qualitative Inquiry*, 10: 421–440.

Papathomas, A., & Lavallee, D. (2010). Athlete experiences of disordered eating in sport. *Qualitative Research in Sport, Exercise and Health*, 2: 354–370.

Paradis, E. (2012). Boxers, briefs or bras? Bodies, gender and change in the boxing gym. *Body and Society*, 18: 82–109.

Partington, E., Partington, S., Fishwick, L., & Allin, L. (2005). Mid-life nuances and negotiations: Narrative maps and the social construction of mid-life in sport and physical activity. *Sport, Education and Society*, 10: 85–99.

Patton, M. (1990). *Qualitative evaluation and research methods*. London: Sage.

Pearson, G. (2009). The researcher as hooligan. *International Journal of Social Research Methodology*, 12: 244–255.

Perrier, M-J., & Kirkby, J. (2013). Taming the 'Dragon': Using voice recognition software for transcription in disability research within sport and exercise psychology. *Qualitative Research in Sport, Exercise and Health*, 5: 103–108.

Phoenix, C. (2010a). Auto-photography in aging studies: Exploring issues of identity construction in mature bodybuilders. *Journal of Aging Studies*, 24: 167–180.

Phoenix, C. (2010b). Seeing the world of physical culture: The potential of visual methods for qualitative research in sport and exercise. *Qualitative Research in Sport, Exercise and Health*, 2: 93–108.

Phoenix, C., & Griffin, M. (2012). Narratives at work: What can stories of older athletes do? *Ageing and Society*, 33: 243–266.

Phoenix, C., & Smith, B. (2011). Telling a (good?) counterstory of aging: Natural bodybuilding meets the narrative of decline. *The Journals of Gerontology Series B: Psychological Sciences and Social Sciences*, 66: 628–639.

Phoenix, C., & Sparkes, A. (2006). Young athletic bodies and narrative maps of aging. *Journal of Aging Studies*, 20: 107–121.

Phoenix, C., & Sparkes, A. (2007). Sporting bodies, ageing, narrative mapping and young team athletes: An analysis of possible selves. *Sport, Education and Society*, 12: 1–17.

Phoenix, C., & Sparkes, A. (2008). Athletic bodies and aging in context: The narrative construction of experienced and anticipated selves in time. *Journal of Aging Studies*, 22: 211–221.

Phoenix, C., & Sparkes, A. (2009). Being Fred: Big stories, small stories and the accomplishment of a positive aging identity. *Qualitative Research*, 9: 219–236.

Pickard, A. & Bailey, R. (2009). Crystallising experiences among young elite dancers. *Sport, Education and Society*, 14: 165–181.

Pike, L. (2011). The active aging agenda, old folk devils and a new moral panic. *Sociology of Sport Journal*, 28: 209–225.

Pink, S. (2007). *Doing visual ethnography* (2nd ed.). London: Sage.

Pitney, W., & Parker, J. (2009). *Qualitative research in physical activity and the health professions*. Champaign, IL: Human Kinetics.

Plummer, K. (2001). *Documents of life 2*. London: Sage.

Poizat, S., Saury, G., & Durand, M. (2006). A ground theory of elite male table tennis players' activity during matches. *The Sport Psychologist*, 20: 58–73.

Post, P., & Wrisberg, C. (2012). A phenomenological investigation of gymnasts' lived experience of imagery. *Sport Psychologist,* 24: 98–121.

Pridgeon, L., & Grogan, S. (2012). Understanding exercise adherence and dropout: An interpretative phenomenological analysis of men and women's accounts of gym attendance and non-attendance. *Qualitative Research in Sport, Exercise and Health*, 4: 382–399.

Purdy, L., Potrac, P., & Jones, R. (2008). Power, consent and resistance: An autoethnography of competitive rowing. *Sport, Education and Society*, 13: 319–336.

Randall, W., & Phoenix, C. (2009). The problem with truth in qualitative interviews: reflections from a narrative perspective. *Qualitative Research in Sport, Exercise and Health*, 1: 125–140.

Ravn, S., & Ploug Hansen, H. (2012). How to explore dancers' sense experiences? A study of how multi-sited fieldwork and phenomenology can be combined. *Qualitative Research in Sport, Exercise and Health.* DOI: 1080/2159676X.2012.712991.

Richards, L. (2005). *Handling qualitative data*. London: Sage.

Richardson, L. (2000). Writing: A method of inquiry. In N. Denzin & Y. Lincoln (Eds.), *Handbook of qualitative research* (2nd ed., pp. 923–948). London: Sage.

Richardson, L., & St. Pierre, E. (2005). Writing: A method of inquiry. In N. Denzin & Y. Lincoln (Eds.), *Handbook of qualitative research* (3rd ed., pp. 959–978). London: Sage.

Richardson, S., Andersen, M., & Morris, T. (2008). *Overtraining athletes: Personal journeys in sport*. Champaign, IL: Human Kinetics.

Riessman, K. (2008). *Narrative methods for the human sciences*. London: Sage.

Ruddin, L. (2006). You can generalize stupid! Social scientists, Bent Flyvbjerg, and case study methodology. *Qualitative Inquiry*, 12: 797–812.

Ryba, T., Haapanen, S., Mosek., S. & Ng, K. (2012). Toward a conceptual understanding of acute cultural adaption: A preliminary examination of aca in female swimming. *Qualitative Research in Sport, Exercise and Health*, 4: 80–97.

Saldaña, J. (2011a). *The coding manual for qualitative researchers*. London: Sage.

Saldaña, J. (2011b). *Ethnotheatre: Research from page to stage*. Walnut Creek, CA: Left Coast Press.

Sands, R. (2002). *Sports ethnography*. Champaign, IL: Human Kinetics.

Sanjek, R. (1991). The ethnographic present. *Man: The Journal of the Royal Anthropological Institute*, 26: 609–628.

Scheurich, R. (1997). *Research method in the postmodern*. Lewes: Falmer Press.

Schwandt, T. (1997). *Qualitative inquiry: A dictionary of terms.* London: Sage.

Schwandt, T. (2001). *Dictionary of qualitative inquiry* (2nd ed.). Thousand Oaks, CA: Sage.

Scott-Dixon, K. (2008) Big girls don't cry: Fitness, fatness and the production of feminist knowledge. *Sociology of Sport Journal,* 25: 22–47.

Scott, S. (2010). How to look good (nearly) naked: The performative regulation of the swimmer's body. *Body and Society,* 16: 143–168.

Sheridan, J., Chamberlain, K., & Dupuis, A. (2011). Timelining: Visualizing experience. *Qualitative Research,* 11: 552–569.

Shilling, C., & Bunsell, T. (2009). The female bodybuilder as gender outlaw. *Qualitative Research in Sport, Exercise and Health,* 1: 141–159.

Silverman, D. (2000). *Doing qualitative research.* London: Sage.

Singer, J., & Cunningham, G. (2012). A case study of the diversity culture of an American university athletic department: Perceptions of senior level administrators. *Sport, Education and Society,* 17: 647–669.

Slater, M., Spray, C., & Smith, B. (2012). 'You're only as good as your weakest link': Implicit theories of golf ability. *Psychology of Sport and Exercise,* 13: 280–290.

Smith, A., & Stewart, B. (2012). Body perceptions and health behaviours on an online bodybuilding community. *Qualitative Health Research,* 22: 971–985.

Smith, B. (2008). Imagining being disabled through playing sport: The body and alterity as limits to imagining others' lives. *Sport, Ethics and Philosophy,* 2: 142–157.

Smith, B. (2010). Narrative inquiry: Ongoing conversations and questions for sport and exercise psychology research. *International Review of Sport and Exercise Psychology,* 3: 87–107.

Smith, B. (2013a). Disability, sport, and men's narratives of health: A qualitative study. *Health Psychology,* 32: 110–119.

Smith, B. (2013b). Sporting spinal cord injuries, social relations, and rehabilitation narratives: An ethnographic creative non-fiction of becoming disabled through sport. *Sociology of Sport Journal,* 30: 132–152.

Smith, B. (in press). Artificial persons and the academy: A story. In N. Short. L. Turner & A. Grant (Eds.). *British contemporary autoethnography.* Rotterdam: Sense Publishers.

Smith, B., Allen Collinson, J., Phoenix, C., Brown, D., & Sparkes, A. (2009). Dialogue, monologue, and boundary crossing within research encounters: A performative narrative analysis. *International Journal of Sport and Exercise Psychology,* 7: 342–358.

Smith, B., & Sparkes, A. (2002). Men, sport, spinal cord injury, and the construction of coherence: Narrative practice in action. *Qualitative Research,* 2: 143–171.

Smith, B., & Sparkes, A. (2004). Men, sport, and spinal cord injury: An analysis of metaphors and narrative types. *Disability and Society,* 19: 613–626.

Smith, B., & Sparkes, A. (2005). Men, sport, spinal cord injury, and narratives of hope. *Social Science and Medicine,* 61: 1095–1105.

Smith, B., & Sparkes, A. (2006). Narrative inquiry in psychology: exploring the tensions within. *Qualitative Research in Psychology,* 3: 169–192.

Smith, B., & Sparkes, A. (2008a). Contrasting perspectives on narrating self and identities: An invitation to dialogue. *Qualitative Research*, 8: 5–35.

Smith, B., & Sparkes, A. (2008b). Changing bodies, changing narratives and the consequences of tellability: A case study of becoming disabled through sport. *Sociology of Health and Illness*, 30: 217–236.

Smith, B., & Sparkes, A. (2009a). Narrative inquiry in sport and exercise psychology: What can it mean, and why might we do it? *Psychology of Sport and Exercise*, 10: 1–11.

Smith, B., & Sparkes, A. (2009b). Narrative analysis and sport and exercise psychology: Understanding lives in diverse ways. *Psychology of Sport and Exercise*, 10: 279–288.

Smith, B., & Sparkes, A. (2011). Exploring multiple responses to a chaos narrative. *Health: An Interdisciplinary Journal for the Study of Health, Illness and Medicine*, 15: 38–53.

Smith, B., & Sparkes, A. (2012). Narrative analysis in sport and physical culture. In K. Young & M. Atkinson (Eds.), *Qualitative research on sport and physical culture* (pp. 79–101). Bingley, UK: Emerald Group Publishing Ltd.

Smith, J. (1989). *The nature of social and educational inquiry: Empiricism versus interpretation*. Norwood, NJ: Ablex Publishing Corporation.

Smith, J. (1993). *After the demise of empiricism: The problem of judging social and educational inquiry*. Norwood, NJ: Ablex Publishing Corporation.

Smith, J. (2011). Evaluating the contribution of interpretative phenomenological analysis. *Health Psychology Review*, 5: 9–27.

Smith, J., & Deemer, D. (2000). The problem of criteria in the age of relativism. In N. Denzin & Y. Lincoln (Eds.), *Handbook of qualitative research* (2nd ed., pp. 877–896). London: Sage.

Smith, J., Flowers, P., & Larkin, M. (2009). *Interpretive phenomenological analysis: Theory, methods, research*. London: Sage.

Smith, J., & Hodkinson, P. (2005). Relativism, criteria and politics. In N. Denzin & Y. Lincoln (Eds.), *Handbook of qualitative research* (3rd ed., pp. 915–932). London: Sage.

Smith, J., & Hodkinson, P. (2009). Challenging neorealism: A response to Hammersley'. *Qualitative Inquiry*, 15: 30–39.

Smith, J., Jarman, A., & Osborn, M. (1999). Doing interpretive phenomenological analysis. In M. Murray & K. Chamberlain (Eds.), *Qualitative health psychology* (pp. 218–240). London: Sage.

Smith, J., & Osborn, M. (2003). Interpretive phenomenological analysis'. In J. Smith (Ed.). *Qualitative psychology: A practical guide to research methods* (pp. 51–80). London: Sage.

Soundy, A., Smith, B., Cressy, F., & Webb, L. (2010). The experience of spinal cord injury: Using Frank's narrative types to enhance physiotherapy undergraduates' understanding. *Physiotherapy*, 96: 52–58.

Sparkes, A. (1992). The paradigms debate: An extended review and a celebration of difference'. In A. Sparkes (Ed.), *Research in physical education and sport: Exploring alternative visions* (pp. 9–60). London: Falmer Press.

Sparkes, A. (1996) 'The fatal flaw': A narrative of the fragile body-self. *Qualitative Inquiry*, 2: 463–495.

Sparkes, A. (1998). Validity in qualitative inquiry and the problem of criteria: Implications for sport psychology. *The Sport Psychologist*, 12: 363–386.

Sparkes, A. (1999). Exploring body narratives. *Sport, Education and Society*, 4: 17–30.

Sparkes, A. (2000). Autoethnographies and narratives of self: Reflections on criteria in action. *Sociology of Sport Journal*, 17: 21–43.

Sparkes, A. (2002a). *Telling tales in sport and physical activity: A qualitative journey*. Champaign, IL: Human Kinetics Press.

Sparkes, A. (2002b). Autoethnography: Self-indulgence or something more? In A. Bochner & C. Ellis (Eds.), *Ethnographically speaking: Autoethnography, literature, and aesthetics* (pp. 209–232). London: Altamira Press.

Sparkes, A. (2002c). Fictional representations: On difference, choice, and risk. *Sociology of Sport Journal*, 19: 1–24.

Sparkes, A. (2003a). Bodies, identities, selves: autoethnographic fragments and reflections. In J. Denison & P. Markula (Eds.), *'Moving writing': Crafting movement and sport research* (pp. 51–76). New York: Peter Lang.

Sparkes, A. (2003b). From performance to impairment: A patchwork of embodied memories. In J. Evans, B. Davies & J. Wright (Eds.), *Body knowledge and control* (pp. 157–172). London: Routledge.

Sparkes, A. (2004). Bodies, narratives, selves and autobiography: The example of Lance Armstrong. *Journal of Sport and Social Issues*, 28: 397–428.

Sparkes, A. (2005). Narrative analysis: exploring the *whats* and *hows* of personal stories. In I. Holloway (Ed.), *Qualitative research in health care* (pp. 191–209). Buckingham, UK: Open University Press.

Sparkes, A. (2007). Embodiment, academics, and the audit culture: A story seeking consideration'. *Qualitative Research*, 7: 519–548.

Sparkes, A. (2008). Sport and physical education: Embracing new forms of representation. In J. Knowles & A. Cole (Eds.), *Handbook of arts in qualitative research* (pp. 653–664). London: Sage.

Sparkes, A. (2009a). Ethnography and the senses: Challenges and possibilities. *Qualitative Research in Sport, Exercise and Health*, 1: 21–35.

Sparkes, A. (2009b). Novel ethnographic representations and the dilemmas of judgment. *Ethnography and Education*, 4: 303–321.

Sparkes, A. (2012) Fathers and sons: In bits and pieces. *Qualitative Inquiry*, 18: 167–178.

Sparkes, A. (2013) Qualitative research in sport, exercise and health in the era of neoliberalism, audit, and new public management: Understanding the conditions for the (im)possibilities of a new paradigm dialogue. *Qualitative Research in Sport, Exercise & Health*, DOI: 10.1080/2159676X.2013.79.

Sparkes, A., Batey, J., & Owen, G. (2012). The muscled self and the dynamics of shame and pride: A bodybuilding life history. In A. Locks & N. Richardson (Eds.). *Critical readings in bodybuilding* (pp. 107–121). London: Routledge.

Sparkes, A., Brown, D., & Partington, E. (2010). The 'jock body' and the social construction of space: The performance and positioning of cultural identity. *Space and Culture*, 13, 333–347.

Sparkes, A., & Douglas, K. (2007). Making the case for poetic representations: An example in action. *The Sport Psychologist*, 21: 170–189.

Sparkes, A., Nilges, L., Swan, P. & Dowling, F. (2003). Poetic representations in sport and physical activity: Insider perspectives. *Sport, Education and Society*, 8: 153–177.

Sparkes, A., & Partington, E. & Brown, D. (2007). Bodies as bearers of value: The transmission of jock culture via the 'Twelve Commandments'. *Sport, Education and Society*, 12: 295–316.

Sparkes, A., & Partington, S. (2003). Narrative practice and its potential contribution to sport psychology: The example of flow. *The Sport Psychologist*, 17: 292–317.

Sparkes, A., Pérez-Samaniego, V., & Smith, B. (2012). Social comparison processes, narrative mapping, and their shaping of the cancer experience: A case study of an elite athlete. *Health: An Interdisciplinary Journal for the Study of Health, Illness and Medicine*, 16, 467–488.

Sparkes, A., & Smith, B. (2002). Sport, spinal cord injuries, embodied masculinities and the dilemmas of narrative identity. *Men and Masculinities*, 4: 258–285.

Sparkes, A., & Smith, B. (2003). Men, sport, spinal cord injury and narrative time. *Qualitative Research*, 3: 295–320.

Sparkes, A., & Smith, B. (2005). When narratives matter: men, sport, and spinal cord injury. *Journal of Medical Humanities*, 31: 81–88.

Sparkes, A., & Smith, B. (2008a) Men, spinal cord injury, memories, and the narrative performance of pain. *Disability and Society*, 23: 679–690.

Sparkes, A., & Smith, B. (2008b). Narrative constructionist inquiry. In J. Holstein & J. Gubrium (Eds.), *Handbook of constuctionist research* (pp. 295–314). New York: Guildford Publications Inc.

Sparkes, A., & Smith, B. (2009) Judging the quality of qualitative inquiry: Criteriology and relativism in action. *Psychology of Sport and Exercise*, 10: 491–497.

Sparkes, A., & Smith, B. (2011). Inhabiting different bodies over time: Narrative and pedagogical challenges. *Sport, Education and Society*, 16: 357–370.

Sparkes, A., & Smith, B. (2012a). Narrative analysis as an embodied engagement with the lives of others. In J. Gubrium & J. Holstein (Eds.), *Varieties of narrative analysis* (pp. 53–73). London: Sage.

Sparkes A., & Smith, B. (2012b). Embodied research methodologies and the senses in sport and physical culture: A fleshing out of problems and possibilities. In K. Young & M. Atkinson (Eds.), *Qualitative research on sport and physical culture* (pp. 169–192). Bingley, UK: Emerald Group Publishing Ltd.

Spencer, D. (2011). *Ultimate fighting and embodiment: Violence, gender and mixed martial arts*. London: Taylor and Francis.

Spencer, D. (2012). Narratives of despair and loss: Pain, injury and masculinity in the sport of mixed martial arts. *Qualitative Research in Sport, Exercise and Health*, 4: 117–137.

Stake, R. (1995). *The art of case study research*. London: Sage.

Stake, R. (2005). Qualitative case studies. In N. Denzin & Y. Lincoln (Eds.), *Handbook of qualitative research* (3rd ed., pp. 443–466). London: Sage.

Steiner, L. (2009). Feminist media ethics. In L. Wilkins & C. Christians (Eds.), *The handbook of mass media ethics* (pp. 366–381). New York: Routledge.

266

Stevens, L. & Andersen, M. (2007). Transference and countertransference in sport psychology service delivery: Part II. Two case studies on the erotic. *Journal of Applied Sport Psychology*, 19: 270–287.

Stewart, C., Smith, B., & Sparkes, A. (2011). Sporting autobiographies of illness and the role of metaphor. *Sport in Society*, 14: 581–597.

Stone, B. (2009). Running man. *Qualitative Research in Sport, Exercise and Health*, 1: 67–71.

Strauss, A., & Corbin, J. (1998). *Basics of qualitative research: Grounded theory procedures and techniques* (2nd ed.). Thousand Oaks, CA: Sage.

Sugden, J. (2012). Truth or dare: Examining the perils, pains and pitfalls of investigative methodologies in the sociology of sport. In K. Young & M. Atkinson (Eds.), *Qualitative research on sport and physical culture* (pp. 233–252). Bingley, UK: Emerald Group Publishing Ltd.

Sykes, H. (2006). Queering theories of sexuality in sport studies. In J. Caudwell (Ed.), *Sport, sexualities and queer/theory* (pp. 13–32). London: Routledge.

Sykes, H., Chapman, J., & Swedberg, A. (2006). Performed ethnography. In D. Andrews, D. Mason & M. Silk (Eds.), *Qualitative methods in sports studies* (pp. 185–202). Oxford: Berg.

Tamminen, K., Holt, N., & Neely, K. (2013). Exploring adversity and the potential for growth among elite female athletes. *Psychology of Sport and Exercise,* 14: 28–36.

Tawse, H., Bloom, G., Sabiston, C., & Reid, G. (2012). The role of coaches of wheelchair rugby in the development of athletes with spinal cord injury. *Qualitative Research in Sport, Exercise and Health*, 4: 206–225.

Thompson, C., & Andersen, M. (2012). moving toward buddhist psychotherapy in sport: A case study. *The Sport Psychologist*, 26: 624–653.

Thorpe, H. (2008). Foucault, technologies of the self and the media: Discourses of femininity in snowboarding cultures. *Journal of Sport and Social Issues*, 32: 199–229.

Thorpe, H. (2010). Bourdieu, gender reflexivity, and physical culture: A case of masculinities in the snowboarding field. *Journal of Sport and Social Issues*, 34: 176–214.

Thorpe, H. (2011). *Snowboarding bodies in theory and practice*. Basingstoke: Palgrave Macmillan.

Thorpe, H. (2012). The ethnographic interview in the sports field: Towards a postmodern sensibility. In K. Young & M. Atkinson (Eds.). *Qualitative research on sport and physical culture* (pp. 51–78). Bingley, UK: Emerald Group Publishing Ltd.

Tilley, E., & Woodthorpe, K. (2011). Is it the end for anonymity as we know it? A critical examination of the ethical principle of anonymity in the context of 21st century demands on the qualitative researcher. *Qualitative Research*, 11: 197–212.

Tolich, M. (2010). A critique of current practice: Ten foundational Guidelines for Autoethnographers. *Qualitative Health Research*, 20: 1599–1610.

Tracey, J. (2011). Benefits and usefulness of a personal motivation video: A case study of a professional mountain bike rider. *Journal of Applied Sport Psychology*, 23: 308–325.

Tracy, S. (2010). Qualitative quality: Eight 'big tent' criteria for excellent qualitative research. *Qualitative Inquiry*, 16: 837–851.

Tulle, E. (2008). *Ageing, the body and social change: Running in later life*. Basingstoke: Palgrave Macmillan.

Vagle, M. (2011). Validity as intended: 'bursting forth toward' bridling in phenomenological research. *International Journal of Qualitative Studies in Education*, 22: 585–605.

Van Maanen, J. (1988). *Tales from the field: On writing ethnography*. Chicago: University of Chicago Press.

Vannini, P., Waskul, D., & Gottschalk, S. (2012). *The senses in self, society, and culture*. London: Routledge.

Vaughn, B., & Daniel, S. (2012). Conceptualizing validity. In G. Tenenbaum, R. Eklund & A. Kamata (Eds). *Measurement in sport and exercise psychology* (pp. 33–39). Champaign, IL: Human Kinetics.

Wacquant, L. (2004). *Body and soul: Notebooks of an Apprentice boxer*. New York: Oxford University Press.

Wagstaff, C., Fletcher, D., & Hanton. S. (2012). Positive organizational psychology in sport: An ethnography of organizational functioning in a national sport organization. *Journal of Applied Sport Psychology*, 24: 26–47.

Waldron, J., Lynn, Q., & Krane, V. (2011). Duct tape, icy hot and paddles: Narratives of initiation onto US male sport teams. *Sport, Education and Society*, 16: 111–125.

Walford, G. (2005). Research ethical guidelines and anonymity. *International Journal of Research and Method in Education*, 28: 83–93.

Walsh, R., & Koelsch, L. (2012). Building across fault lines in qualitative research. *The Humanist Psychologist*, 40: 380–390.

Watson, C. (2011). Staking a small claim for fictional narratives in social and educational research. *Qualitative Research*, 11: 395–408.

Way, A., Jones, M., & Slater, M. (2012). Exploring training adherence in elite school-age athletes. *Qualitative Research in Sport, Exercise and Health*, 4: 154–171.

Weber, J., & Barker-Ruchti, N. (2012). Bending, flirting, floating, flying: A critical analysis of female figures in 1970s gymnastics photographs. *Sociology of Sport Journal*, 29: 22–41.

Weed, M. (2009a). The structure of (social) scientific contradictions: A comment on the problem of paradigmatic behaviour by social scientists. *Qualitative Research in Sport and Exercise*, 1: 312–321.

Weed, M. (2009b). Research quality considerations for grounded theory research in exercise and sport psychology. *Psychology of Sport and Exercise*, 10: 502–510.

Weed, M. (2010). A qualitative debate on grounded theory in sport and exercise psychology? A commentary on potential areas for future debate. *Psychology of Sport and Exercise*, 11: 414–418.

Weissensteiner, J., Abernethy, B., & Farrow, D. (2009). Towards the development of a conceptual model of expertise in cricket batting: A grounded theory approach. *Journal of Applied Sport Psychology*, 21: 276–292.

West, J., Bill, K., & Martin, L. (2010). What constitutes research ethics in sport and exercise science? *Research Ethics Review*, 6: 147–153.

Whittemore, R., Chase, S., & Mandle, C. (2001). Validity in qualitative research. *Qualitative Health Research*, 11: 522–537.

Wickson, F., Carew, A., & Russell, A. (2006). Transdisciplinary research: Characteristics, quandaries and quality. *Futures*, 38: 1046–1059.

Wiggins, S., & Potter, J. (2008). Discursive psychology. In C. Willig & W. Stainton-Rogers (Eds.), *Handbook of qualitative research in psychology* (pp. 73–90). London: Sage.

Willig, C. (2004). *Introducing qualitative research in psychology*. Milton Keynes: Open University Press.

Woike, B. (2008). The state of the story in personality psychology. *Social and Personality Psychology Compass*, 2: 434–443.

Wolcott, H. (1990). *Writing up qualitative research*. London: Sage.

Wolcott, H. (1994). *Transforming qualitative data*. London: Sage.

Wolcott, H. (1995). *The art of fieldwork*. London: AltaMira Press.

Wolcott, H. (1999). *Ethnography: A way of seeing*. London: Sage.

Wolcott, H. (2002). *Sneaky kid and its aftermath: Ethics and intimacy in fieldwork*. Walnut Creek, CA: AltaMira Press.

Wolcott, H. (2010). *Ethnography lessons: A primer*. Walnut Creek, CA: Left Coast Press.

Yin, R. (1989). *Case study research: Design and methods*. London: Sage.

INDEX

270

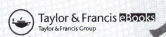

Printed in Great Britain
by Amazon

47723671R00165